MIRACLE MEDICINE HERBS

MIRACLE MEDICINE HERBS

Richard M. Lucas

PARKER PUBLISHING COMPANY
West Nyack, New York 10995

10 9 8 7 6 5 4

10 9 8 7 6 5 4 3 2 (PBK)

Library of Congress Cataloging-in-Publication Data

Lucas, Richard Melvin.
  Miracle medicine herbs / Richard M. Lucas.
    p. cm.

  Includes index.
    ISBN 0-13-585142-4 (case).—ISBN 0-13-585134-3 (paper)
    1. Herbs—Therapeutic use.   I. Title.
RM666.H33L79 1990
615′ .321—dc20   90-22314
                                                        CIP

ISBN 0-13-585142-4

ISBN 0-13-585134-3 (PBK)

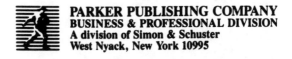

PARKER PUBLISHING COMPANY
BUSINESS & PROFESSIONAL DIVISION
A division of Simon & Schuster
West Nyack, New York 10995

Printed in the United States of America

Other Books by the Author

Nature's Medicines: The Folklore, Romance, and Value of Herbal Remedies

Common and Uncommon Uses of Herbs for Healthful Living

Secrets of the Chinese Herbalists

The Magic of Herbs in Daily Living

Magic Herbs for Arthritis, Rheumatism, and Related Ailments

Herbal Health Secrets from Europe and Around the World

ABOUT THE AUTHOR

Richard Lucas has devoted three decades to the collection, research, and study of literature pertaining to the background, history, and scientific evaluation of the medicinal use of herbs. During this time he contacted and became friends with medical herbalists the world over who generously shared their knowledge, which was carefully recorded and compiled. With the recent development of scientific interest and research in plant medicine, Lucas began contacting numerous laboratories, foundations, pharmacologists, and medical doctors in many countries of the world to learn their opinions on herbal health care. Through their combined knowledge and his own extensive experience and research, Lucas has produced this invaluable, easy-to-follow treatment guide to herbal remedies for a wide range of ailments.

INTRODUCTION

Some of the world's greatest healing agents were derived from the plant kingdom. "It must be remembered," wrote G. Scott Elliot, M.A., B.Sc., Fellow of the Geographical Society, that aborigines "were true experimentalists. They made discoveries which have been of infinite service to mankind. We remember the men like Harvey, Lister, and Pasteur but we never think of the Indian who discovered quinine."

Elliot is referring to the aborigines of South America who used the bark of a Peruvian tree for the treatment of malaria. This tree was named *Chincona* after the wife of a Spanish viceroy (Count de Chincon) who, in about 1638, was cured of fever by its use. In Europe its reputation as a remedy for malaria became so great that the powdered bark was often sold for its weight in gold. However, it was not until almost 200 years later that scientists isolated quinine, a substance which has proved invaluable as an effective treatment of malaria, from the bark.

The herb Ma-huang has been used by the Chinese for thousands of years as a remedy for bronchial spasms, asthmatic attacks, coughs, and similar disorders. Scientists found that the plant contained a substance called *ephedrine*, and physicians soon began prescribing it for pulmonary complaints just as the Chinese have been doing for countless centuries.

Other examples of plant substances discovered and subsequently used by the medical profession include digitalis (heart medication), curare (local anesthetic), morphine (powerful pain killer), and reserpine (tranquilizer), to name just a few.

Present-day scientists are finding that the number of herbs which have supplied such valuable medicines over the past years is just the tip of the iceberg. Researchers are once again investigating many of the plants used as folk remedies, and the results are rewarding. For example:

- The early Greeks, Chinese, Romans, Egyptians, and Hindus claimed that garlic effectively treats intestinal disorders, skin disease, respiratory ailments, and many other health problems. Scientific studies have demonstrated that garlic attacks more than 23 types of bacteria as well as 70 kinds of fungi including *Candida albicans*. Clinical experiments conducted in the U.S.,

Japan, and other countries have shown that adequate amounts of garlic in the diet may protect against some forms of cancer.

• The use of the herb milk thistle is an old folk remedy for treating liver disorders. In recent years clinical studies have demonstrated that an extract of the herb regenerates the liver. Its use was also found effective in preventing, reversing, or curing many liver diseases.

• Propolis is a sticky resinous substance collected by bees from the bark or leaf buds of trees. Centuries ago it was cited in various herb books as a treatment for abscesses, blood and skin disorders, catarrh, and other ailments. Scientist K. Lund Aagaard of Denmark reported that tests on thousands of volunteers have shown that propolis totally or partially cures bacterial and viral infections of the eyes, mouth, throat, nose, and intestines as well as stomach complaints and numerous skin diseases. Studies by other scientists have also reported many remarkable healing effects with its use.

Herbalism is rapidly returning to public favor. Thinking men and women everywhere are finding their way back to health through proper nutrition, adequate sleep, a positive mental attitude, and the use of nature's medicines. In this book you have at your fingertips a large selection of herb remedies for coping with a wide range of ailments. Along with ample coverage of recipes which can be prepared at home, this book presents information about herbal products sold on the market in the form of fluid extracts, tinctures, and so on. Most health food stores carry an excellent variety of herbs and herbal products, but if your local store does not supply them all you can write directly to the mail order firms I've listed for your convenience at the back of this book.

In Chapter 9 you'll read of a large-scale trial in which a certain herbal ointment was used for numerous skin conditions. Over 500 medical specialists participated in the study. The trial involved more than 4,000 patients with inflammatory skin conditions (e.g., dermatitis, abscesses, varicose ulcers of the legs, herpes simplex, various forms of eczema, burns, skin wounds). The overall success rate of 85% was highly significant.

In Chapter 1 you'll read about a remarkable herb, scientifically tested, which builds energy and endurance, improves eyesight and sleep, increases bodily resistance to many diseases, and has a positive effect against most types of acute and chronic stress.

In Chapter 8 you'll learn of an herbal extract which has demonstrated beneficial effects on different parts of the circulatory and nervous systems. It has been recommended as a supplement to resist the effects of premature aging, and, for individuals with symptoms of aging such as short-term memory loss, inattentiveness, and senility, to reduce its effects.

Other chapters cover problems such as PMS (premenstrual syndrome), headaches, bowel complaints, respiratory ailments, liver and gallbladder problems, arthritis, ulcers, and many other disorders. You'll find impressive case histories describing how people achieved remarkable healing benefits from the use of an herb remedy. Consider the following, which are just a few of many examples:

- For years a woman suffered from varicose veins and leg ulcers. She finally had the vein in her left leg stripped, but after a month or so it began to swell again.

  Then she read of a natural substance derived from the plant kingdom and started taking it every day. She reports: "That was 19 years ago. I have never had any vein trouble since, although I worked in a hospital and was on my feet all day."

- Mr. K. relates the case of a man he met one Christmas Day who was suffering from arthritis. The man was unable to bend over, and his fingers were stiff and enlarged. Mr. K. gave him two bags of a certain herb and told him how to prepare it as a tea. In January he gave him two more, and when he went to visit the man's home in March he found him out in his garden with his wife, weeding. The man stood up, put his arms over his head, then stooped down and touched the ground three times. He showed Mr. K. his nimble fingers and said, "I feel like a kid again." After two months he stopped taking the herb tea.

- Dr. Benjamin Lau reports the case of two young women who developed symptoms of hay fever—sneezing, streamy nasal discharge, and watery itching eyes. The antihistamines prescribed by their own physician brought some relief but caused many unpleasant side effects. Desensitizing shots were of little or no benefit.

  Dr. Lau was then consulted, and he instructed each of the young women to take capsules of a certain herbal product every day. Within three weeks both women were free of hay fever symptoms.

- One man suffered from diverticulitis for over two years. He said that his doctor's treatment was ineffective, so he began using special herb tablets, which brought about a remarkable improvement. He reports, "I can now go out all day without any trouble. I am 81 years old and it is a great relief to feel so good.[2]

- Another man wrote that his wife and her sister tried a special herb product for PMS and were delighted with the beneficial results. He said both women agreed that the herbal formula "works like magic."

You will notice that throughout this book several different herbs are cited for the same health problem. This gives you a variety of remedies to choose from, as one remedy does not always fit the needs of every person (there are too many individual differences, too many variables). In this way you can select the remedy most appropriate to your needs, and if after giving one remedy a sufficient trial it does not help, you can switch to another. This procedure does not guarantee success, of course, but it does increase your chances of finding a remedy that may work for you. Herbs are natural food substances which tend to have a gradual effect, so patience is necessary.

Given the right conditions, your body has the power to heal itself. So whatever your illness may be, do not despair. Good health is part of Nature, and it is unlikely that within her vast storehouse she has not provided the material that can help you.

> And God said, Behold I have given you every herb bearing seed, which is upon the face of all the earth, and every tree, in the which is the fruit of a tree yielding seed; to you it shall be for meat.—*Genesis 1:29*
>
> ...and the fruit thereof shall be for meat, and the leaf thereof for medicine.—*Ezekiel 47:12*

GLOSSARY

TERMS RELATING TO HERBAL THERAPEUTIC ACTION

Some of the terms used in this book refer to the therapeutic action of certain herbs according to reference texts on herbal medicine. The most common ones are defined in this glossary.

Alternative: A vague term to indicate a substance which alters a condition by producing a gradual change toward restoration of health. Alternatives are also known as blood purifiers.

Anodyne: Relieves pain.

Anthelmintic: Destroys or expels intestinal worms.

Antibacterial: Destroys germs.

Antibiotic: Arrests or destroys the growth of microorganisms.

Antidote: Counteracts or destroys the effects of poison or other medicines.

Antiseptic: Checks or prevents putrefaction.

Antispasmodic: Prevents or allays spasms or cramps.

Aphrodisiac: Stimulates the sex organs.

Aromatic: Agents which emit a fragrant smell and produce a pungent taste. Used chiefly to make other medicines more palatable.

Calmative: Produces a mild sedative effect.

Cardiac: Produces an effect on the heart.

Carminative: Expels gas from the stomach, intestines, or bowels.

Cholagogue: Increases the flow of bile and promotes its ejection into the small intestine.

Demulcent: Soothing, bland. Used to relieve internal inflammations. Provides a protective coating and allays irritation of the membranes.

Diaphoretic: Induces perspiration.

Digestant: Aids digestion.

Diuretic: Increases the flow of urine. Used to treat water retention. (Because of their soothing qualities, demulcents are often combined with diuretics when irritation is present.)

Emmenagogue: Encourages the menstrual flow.

Expectorant: Induces expulsion of mucus or phlegm from the throat and bronchial passages.

Febrifuge: Reduces fever.

Hepatic: Produces an effect on the liver.

Mucilaginous: Imparts a soothing quality to inflamed areas.

Nervine: Reduces nervous tension or excitement; nourishes the nervous system.

Nutritive; Nutrient: Nourishing.

Pectoral: Relieves affections of the chest and lungs.

Restorative: Aids in regaining normal vigor.

Sedative: Calms the nerves.

Soporific: Induces sleep.

Specific: An agent or remedy that has a special effect on a particular ailment.

Stimulant: Increases or quickens various functional actions of the system.

Stomachic: Tones the stomach. Also used to stimulate the appetite.

Styptic: Acts as an astringent to arrest external bleeding from superficial cuts, scratches, etc.

Tonic: Invigorates and strengthens the system.

Vermifuge: Expels or destroys worms.

TERMS RELATING TO VARIOUS HERBAL PREPARATION METHODS

Compresses

Compresses are local applications to small areas of the skin and may be used either hot or cold depending on the condition being treated. They are prepared by soaking a clean linen cloth in an herbal decoction or infusion. The excess is then wrung out and the compress applied to the affected part.

When a hot compress begins to cool, it is replaced with a fresh one. A cold compress is replaced once it has become warm and somewhat dry from body heat.

Decoctions

Decoctions are made by boiling herbal substances in water for a certain period of time. Hard materials such as roots, barks, or seeds are usually prepared in this way as they require longer subjection to heat in order to extract their active properties.

Extracts

Extracts are made in a variety of ways depending on the best method by which the plant's properties may be obtained, such as high pressure and evaporation by heat. Extracts are supplied by various health food stores and herb firms.

Fomentations

These are prepared in the same way as a compress but are used on larger areas of the skin. Fomentations are applied as hot as possible without burning and then covered with a dry towel. A hot water bottle may be placed over the towel to retain the heat.

Homeopathic Remedies

The system of homeopathy was founded by Dr. Samuel Hahnemann and has been used in the U.S. since 1832. It is based on the theory and practice that disease is cured by remedies which produce in a healthy person effects similar to the symptoms of the disease in a sick person—*Simila Similibus Curentur*, "like cures like." For example, peeling or eating a raw onion produces a watery discharge from the eyes and nose; therefore the onion is the homeopathic remedy for the type of common cold characterized by these symptoms.

Homeopathic remedies are drawn only from natural sources. They are prepared in the form of tiny tablets, pellets, or tinctures. Each remedy undergoes a process of successive dilutions called *potentizing*. These potencies are microscopic—for example, one part of the remedy to 99 parts of the diluted substance (milk sugar). They are labeled 1x, 3x, 6x, and so on. The number before the x reveals how many times the basic ingredient has been diluted and potentized. They can go as high as 1/100th part remedy in ratio to the inert substance, or much higher. The higher the number, the lower the amount of the original remedy remains and the most potent the possible beneficial effects. For home use the potencies commonly employed are either 3x, 6x, 12x, and sometimes 30x.

Homeopathic physicians consider the patient as a whole—his or her emotional and mental states and physical condition as well.

Infusions

Infusions are frequently called *teas*. Usually the softer substances of the herb, such as the blossoms or leaves, are prepared as infusions.

Boiling water is poured over the herb, and the solution is allowed to steep (stand) for a certain amount of time. Infusions are never allowed to boil.

Poultices

Poultices are used locally to relieve inflammation or to cleanse and heal an affected area. They may be applied warm at body temperature or hot according to the condition being treated.

Poultices may be prepared with herb leaves or herb powder. If the leaves are used, they are steeped in hot water and spread between two pieces of cloth. This is applied to the affected part and then covered with a dry towel. If a hot poultice is used, the towel should be covered with a hot water bottle to retain the heat. From time to time the poultice is moistened with water, as it should not be allowed to become dry. Every three or four hours the poultice is replaced with a fresh one, and the process is continued until results are achieved. However, some conditions require more frequent poulticing.

The herb in powder form is often used in place of the leaves. Enough of the herb powder for several poultices is placed in a double boiler. Hot water is stirred into the powder until it attains the consistency of a paste. The mixture is then spread inside a folded cloth, and the same procedure is followed as with the leaves.

Tinctures

Tinctures are spirituous preparations made with pure or diluted alcohol. They are employed because some herbs will not yield their properties to water alone or may be rendered useless by applications of heat. In other instances, an herb will more readily impart its active principles when prepared as a tincture.

Tinctures are available from many health food stores and herb firms.

TABLE OF CONTENTS

CHAPTER 1

HERBS FOR STRENGTHENING THE IMMUNE SYSTEM

The importance of building a strong, healthy immune system has received much attention lately. Many illnesses so prevalent in the world today, such as cancer, Epstein-Barr, candidiasis, and chronic intestinal infections are now believed to be immune-related disorders.

Overcoming dreaded diseases has long been a struggle in the field of medicine, but now there is a great potential for using the body's own defense system to win the battle.

A Brief Word about How the Immune System Functions

The health of the immune system depends on the harmonious interaction of all the components which permit the body to identify the presence of abnormal or foreign substances, to eliminate damaged and worn-out body cells, and to destroy abnormal or mutant cells such as cancer. It is also concerned with the elimination of allergens and the neutralization of pollution.

Modern research has also shown that the immune system interacts with other systems of the body including the hormonal and nervous systems and is not separated from them.

Protector Blood Cells

The white blood cells, the plasma cells, and the macrophages are the protector blood cells of the defense system and are distributed throughout the tissues and organs of the body.

1

Macrophages are believed to produce interferon and to activate the formation of antibodies (interferon and antibodies fight disease organisms and antigens).

The antibody production depends largely on the cooperation of the T- and B-cell systems. Immature white blood cells are attracted from the bloodstream by the influence of the thymus gland, and they mature into different T-cells known as helper T-cells, killer T-cells, and suppressor T-cells. Conversion of the B-cells is believed to occur in the bone marrow.

When the T-cells discover invading foreign substances, they surround and chemically attack them. They can also summon the macrophages to digest the invaders. When the B-cells detect a foreign invader, they produce specific antibodies to neutralize or destroy the intruder. T-cells can also act as helper cells to assist the B-cells in their production of antibodies. Suppressor cells prevent the activity of the defense system from getting out of hand where there may be the risk of the B- or T-cells attacking healthy tissues in the body. However, another danger can occur if the ratio of suppressor to helper cells changes to an excess of suppressors in contrast to the amount present in normal health. In that case, the immune function becomes suppressed and will have difficulty fighting viruses and bacterias.

The cells of the immune system are also called *lymphocytes*.

The Dangers of a Weakened Immune System

Imbalances or a severe disruption of the immune function can result in a vast array of diseases. T-cell defects are associated with recurrent viral infections, as well as fungal infections such as candidiasis. So when the defense system is weakened , not only do infections occur more frequently, but there is the danger of drastic health problems arising (for example, the Acquired Immune Deficiency Syndrome, or AIDS). In the condition of AIDS, it is the T- and B-cell systems that function inadequately.

Some other examples of severe immune deficiency diseases are multiple sclerosis, Epstein-Barr, Graves disease, cystic fibrosis, and certain types of kidney ailments, asthmas, anemias, and allergies.

The Enemies of Immune Strength

Some of the factors leading to a weakened immune system include stress, exposure to environmental toxins, faulty diet, sedentary lifestyle, inadequate sleep, alcohol and tobacco abuse, malabsorption, antibiotics, chemotherapy, birth control pills, cortisone, and other drug therapies.

HERBS FOR ENHANCING THE IMMUNE SYSTEM

Studies have indicated that some of the strongest immune system boosters come from specific healing herbs. A number of these plants are known as adaptogens, which strengthen and normalize the nervous and hormonal systems thereby helping us to adapt to (withstand) the many diverse stresses of modern times. Some also contain antioxidant components which can slow down the cellular aging process and bolster the immune system as well. Others contain the desirable immunostimulating poly-saccharides, which have a broad range of therapeutic activity. For example, they assist the immune system in its fight against invading antigens (bacteria and viruses) and have the potential for fighting cancer. They are also able to relieve the side effects of certain cancer treatments, such as chemotherapy, and to help suppress the metastasis (spreading) of cancer after surgery. A number of other herbs are powerful tonics which strengthen the immune system at a very deep level. They have been known to support T-cell function, activate macrophages, and help rebuild bone marrow reserves.

In short, specific healing herbs have the ability to strengthen and harmonize degenerative body systems. But they cannot do the job alone. Other health practices should be incorporated, such as correct eating habits, nutritional supplements, exercise, adequate sleep, a supportive environment, and a positive mental attitude. (There is irrefutable evidence that what goes on in the mind can affect the immune system.)

The following are some of the most outstanding of the herbal immune enhancers.

ECHINACEA

Botanical Names: *Echinacea angustifolia—Echinacea purpurea*
Common Names: Coneflower, Purple Coneflower

Echinacea is indigenous to North America and Mexico but has been cultivated in Europe. It is a perennial, reaching from 2 to 3 feet in height with thick, rough, hairy leaves. The flower has large spreading purple rays and a disk consisting of purple florets. There are several varieties of this plant family, but the two most effective medicinally are *Echinacea angustifolia* and *Echinacea purpurea*.

Early Medicinal Uses of Echinacea

Echinacea was a popular remedy of the Native Americans, who considered it a universal antidote for snake bites, venomous stings, and septic conditions. Many tribes also used it for treating burns, headaches, enlarged glands, stomach cramps, and toothache.

The first mention of echinacea in a medical journal appeared in a note by Dr. John King in 1887. Its use by other physicians soon followed, and the plant was praised as an excellent blood purifier and alterative, a reputation it enjoys to this day.

Echinacea in Modern Times

Dr. Alfred Vogel of Switzerland, who has taken great interest in herbal medicine, writes:

> During my stay in Mexico, I noted many things which were a useful addition to my knowledge of plants and their properties. There is one special plant which is most used in Mexico and which is well-known to the natives; this is Echinacea. It prevents infection and inflammation in a most remarkable way. It has many friends amongst those who have faith in healing according to the biological method, and it is for this reason that much attention has lately been paid to it in Europe and elsewhere. Echinacea has also proved its worth as an antidote to the unpleasant side effects of penicillin and also in cases where there exists a resistance to penicillin.[1]

The interest in echinacea to which Dr. Vogel refers consists of over 200 in-depth clinical studies conducted over a period of many years. These studies have concluded that echinacea is one of the most effective of the immune enhancing botanicals. It contains compounds found to be antiviral and antibacterial as well as the immunostimulating polysaccharides. It is believed that the antiviral action does not have a direct effect on the viruses but rather that it probably enhances the resistance of the cells to infection.[2]

Echinacea Products

Nearly all the world's scientific studies on echinacea have been conducted with a product known in Europe as Echinacin™. This preparation is derived from the fresh plant juice of *Echinacea purpurea* and has been clinically verified not only as a potent immune booster of the defensive powers of the body but as an effective treatment of many ailments as well. Echinacin has proved of particular value in chronic inflammatory conditions and infections and as a supplementary agent in acute infections. Some forms of arthritis and neuralgia have been relieved with its use, and it has been effectively employed as a supportive measure for dermatological disorders. For over 15 years the product has been sold in Germany for the prophylactic treatment of the flu and for infections.

Echinacin, along with directions for its use , is now available in the U.S. In this country it is sold under the name of Echinace™ (pronounced ek-in-ace).

There are a number of other echinacea products currently available on the market. Some contain a mixture of *Echinacea angustifolia* and *Echinacea purpurea*. These two varieties of the herb have slightly different properties, but both are fine supporters of the immune system. Another product called Echinaforce™ is imported from Switzerland and prepared from both the root and herb of echinacea. Swiss homeopathic immune formulas of echinacea are also available.

Dosages for any of the products will vary according to their strength, so follow the recommendations on the bottle.

ASTRAGALUS

Botanical Name: Astragalus membranaceus and related species
Common Name: Astragali

This perennial herb reaches about 2 feet in height and grows in the northeastern provinces of China. The woody interior of the root is of a yellowish color and has a taste somewhat resembling that of licorice.

Traditional Uses

Astragalus (pronounced as-tra-goo-lus) has been traditionally used in the Orient for thousands of years for debility, anemia, poor appetite, night sweats, weakness during convalescence, lassitude of limbs, and lack of vitality (severely immunosuppressed patients). It was extensively employed as an ingredient in ancient formulas and is mentioned as a superior tonic in *The Pen Tsao Kang Mu* (The General Catalog of Herbs).

Modern Uses

Astragalus is classed as tonic, diuretic, stimulant, and antibacterial. It contains the important polysaccharides and is highly acclaimed as probably the most important of all the deep immune tonics, supporting T-cell function and overall immune strength at a very deep level (bone marrow reserves).[3]

Chinese medical research has demonstrated that the levels of interferon and antibodies increase with the use of astragalus. Its use has also been shown to strengthen vitality, eliminate toxins, promote the healing of damaged tissues, enhance the function of the liver and spleen, protect the liver from chemical damage, and to normalize the blood pressure. As one of the best of the immune boosting agents, astragalus doubled the survival rate of cancer patients when it was administered in addition to chemo- or radiotherapies.

Various Ways of Using Astragalus

- As a tonic root, astragalus is commonly used in Chinese cuisine. It is added to rice or soup stock to strengthen the *chi* (vital force) of the body.

- In order to strengthen its harmonizing effects on the functions of the internal organs and to increase vitality and immune response, astragalus is sometimes processed with honey. One such product contains astragalus root extract with linden honey. It comes in tiny bottles (vials) packed 10 to a carton. One bottle of the extract is taken twice daily, once in the morning and once in the evening. The bottles should be kept in a cool place but not refrigerated. Each bottle should be shaken before using.

- A popular combination of immune enhancing herbs, according to Chinese traditional principles, is known as Astragalus Eight Herbs Formula. It consists of the following botanicals in addition to astragalus: schizandra (energy-tonic—enhances mental activity and physical energy); white atractylodes (immunostimulating agent); ligusticum (used as a tonic when the immune system is failing); codonopsis (considered to contain properties nearly identical to those of ginseng); eleuthero (adaptogen—one of the best tonics and general immune enhancers); ganoderma (contains antitumor properties); licorice (used to enhance and harmonize the ingredients in the Astragalus Eight Herbs Formula).

This formula is available in powder and tablet form. Recommended dosage of the powder is 2 to 3 grams three times daily over a period of several months. The powder may be added to soups, rice, or other foods or prepared as an herbal tea and taken with meals. The effects reportedly include reduced anxiety, more restful sleep, improved liver function, normalization of the blood pressure, and less frequency of infections.

Recommended dosage of the tablet is two to four tablets three times per day. Those using the tablets report reduced incidence of infections, improved energy, and reduction of allergies.

Note. A number of other astragalus products are available on the market. Check with your health food store or herb firm.

GANODERMA

Botanical Name: *Ganoderma lucidium*
Common Names: Reishi, Lingshi

This medicinal mushroom grows wild, primarily on old broadleaf trees. It has a purplish-brown or reddish-brown color and a stalk usually ranging from 2 to 6 inches in length. It is well known in China where it is called lingshi, and very popular in Japan under the name of reishi.

In early Oriental materia-medicas, reishi was listed as a superior medicine to ward off disease, preserve health, and promote longevity. It had been traditionally employed as a *chi* tonic.

Modern Uses

Reishi contains vitamins B_1, B_2, B_3, C, D, and pantothenic acid along with protein, fiber, calcium, phosphorus, and iron. It also contains polysaccharides.

In China, many pharmacological, chemical, and biochemical studies have been conducted with this remarkable mushroom. Results show that reishi meets all qualifications of being an adaptogen and tonic. Its use bolsters the immune system, stimulates health, and improves or prevents allergic conditions and a variety of degenerative and other disease conditions.

Here is a brief summary of the beneficial action of reishi:

- Protects against some types of cancer.
- Increases vitality and strengthens internal organs.
- Relieves neurasthenia and stress.
- Improves conditions of viral hepatitis (70% of all cases with this condition showed marked improvement after taking reishi).
- Protects the liver against chemical damage.
- Helps to normalize body functions.
- Relieves insomnia by enhancing muscle relaxation.

- Improves the coronary arteries.
- Reduces excessive levels of cholesterol in the blood, thus improving circulation. (It has been suggested that since one type of gallstone is formed of cholesterol, the use of reishi extract can reduce the possibility of gallstone formation and may even eliminate existing stones.)

Availability of Reishi

In its wild state reishi is rare, but since it has been successfully cultivated it is available both as a powder and a tablet. However, the most potent form of reishi is the very rare antler form which has many branches and is highest in spores. The cultivated antler form is obtainable either as a powder by itself or combined with powdered shiitake mushroom. The powder may be used as an herbal tea or added to soup or other foods. Directions for taking the tablets are listed on the labels of the bottles.

SHIITAKE

Botanical Name: *Lentinus edodes*
Common Name: Forest Mushroom

The shiitake mushroom is closely related to the reishi and was first discovered growing wild on a Japanese evergreen oak tree. It also grows on other varieties of oaks and is currently cultivated in Japan.

Early Uses

Shiitake has been used in China for centuries. During the Ming Dynasty (1368—1644 A.D.) this remarkable mushroom was added to the diet, not only as a food but also as a remedy for upper respiratory diseases, impaired circulation, liver problems, extreme exhaustion, and weakness. It was also believed to fortify the general health and to prevent premature aging.

Modern Uses

Shiitake is classed as a deep-immune tonic and adaptogen. It contains the polysaccharide *lentinan* which has been studied mostly for its immunostimulating effects and anticancer action. It activates the T-helper cells, the macrophages, and induces interferon production.

One person in Japan reportedly recovered from AIDS after consuming large quantities of shiitake mushroom extract.

In another report which appeared in a Japanese newspaper, we find the following:[4]

> A virus in Japanese mushrooms (shiitake) can be made to produce interferon. Effective in treating cancer, it has been reported in a joint study by the medical department of Kobe University and the Nippon, Kinoko Institute.
>
> Interferon is believed to be capable of fighting off the invasion of virus into cells.
>
> According to Associate Professor Manabu-Takeharu of the University, spherical particles of virus under the cap of the shiitake contain double-stranded RNA, effective not only in restraining the intrusions into the cells but also capable of inducing cells to produce interferon.

Dried shiitake mushrooms can be added to food, or the extract may be taken in tablet form. The properties are similar to reishi, but the latter is more potent.

ELEUTHERO

Botanical Name: *Eleutherococcus senticosis*
Common Names: Siberian Ginseng, Touch-Me-Not, Devil's Bush

This tall shrub is native to various areas of China as well as to the southern regions of the Soviet Far East and belongs to the same plant family as *Panax ginseng*. The shrub blooms in July with violet or yellowish flowers and bears clusters of purple berry-like fruits which ripen in September.

People in olden days named the herb touch-me-not and devil's bush because of its branches, which are spike with thorns. In modern times it is simply called eleuthero, or more commonly Siberian ginseng, as the plant has been tested extensively at the Far Eastern Center of the Siberian Division of the USSR Academy of Sciences.

Eleuthero: A Powerful Adaptogen and Antioxidant

During the past 30 years, over 1,000 scientific studies have been devoted to the adaptogenic effects of eleuthero. As a result, the power of the herb to increase the human body's adaptive capacity to various abnormal physical, biological, chemical, and psychological factors, along with its almost complete nontoxicity, has earned it the title "King of the Adaptogens."

In addition, Soviet researchers have determined that eleuthero also possesses antioxidant action which helps to protect the body against free radical damage. A free radical is a fragment of a molecule that has been torn away from its source and tends to join the body's normal molecules, which it can seriously damage or even cause a chain reaction of molecular destruction. Cells die, enzymes fail to function, energy is reduced, and the body's ability to renew itself and resist or recover from illness is diminished. Antioxidants can almost completely suppress the destructive reactions caused by free radicals.

The Health Benefits of Eleuthero

Clinical findings on eleuthero have established that the herb has a remarkably wide range of therapeutic activity. Here are some examples of its benefits:

- Builds energy and endurance.
- Increases mental and physical work capacity and reflex action.
- Improves circulation, appetite, and sleep.
- Helps in conditions where degeneration of the aging process is noted.
- Improves eyesight, color perception, and hearing.
- Increases bodily resistance to influenza, acute respiratory disease, and other diseases.
- Has a remarkable protective effect against most types of acute and chronic stress.
- Reinforces antitumor immunity.
- Is effective as an adjunct to cancer treatments (retards development of metastases and alleviates the side effects of chemo- and radiation therapies).
- Produces a therapeutic effect in the initial stages of atherosclerosis.

Studies have also shown that eleuthero produces a normalizing effect; for example, reduces a high cholesterol level, increases a low hemoglobin level, lowers elevated sugar content in the blood (mild and moderate cases), normalizes low blood pressure and moderate forms of high blood pressure. Yet this action does not interfere with normal function; that is, it does not in any way disturb normal blood pressure, normal hemo-globin levels, etc.

Case Studies Demonstrate the Benefits of Eleuthero

After extensive clinical tests on laboratory animals had con-clusively demonstrated the beneficial action of eleuthero, the herb's effects were then tested on human subjects. Following are a few examples of the many impressive results which have been reported in Soviet medical writings:

Reduction of Disease Incidence. The properties of ele-uthero in boosting the immune system are apparent from studies in which the incidence of illness and absenteeism was reduced among workers who used the herbal extract. In one study, 1,200 drivers employed at a Russian automobile factory were given eleuthero extract with tea, annually for two months in the spring and autumn for two years. The purpose was to determine whether the extract would increase the drivers' tolerance to the physical and emotional stress produced by the adverse working conditions of noise, exhaust fumes, vibration, and extreme changes of climate. At the completion of the study the incidence of illness among the participants dropped by 20% to 30% while it increased among the workers who did not take the extract.

Two years later another study involved 13,096 employees at the same automobile plant. Eleuthero, in the form of eleuthero sugar, was added to the meals of those participating in the study. The incidence of illness fell by 30% to 35% compared to the group who did not take part in the test.

In other studies, a group of miners took eleuthero extract daily before each work shift for over two months. The incidence of illness fell by 33.3% and by 45.6% regarding the number of disability days.

Functional Nervous Disorders. Patients suffering from nervous exhaustion and nervous emotional disturbances char-acterized by symptoms of depression, chronic insomnia, irrita-bility, anxiety, moodiness, lethargy, and chronic fatigue were treated with a dose of 20 to 40 drops of eleuthero extract three times daily for four to five weeks. In the majority of cases the extract brought about improved sleep and a marked sense of well-being. The normalizing effects were also displayed. Moods of the patients became well balanced, and their interest in life and work improved. Signs of lethargy, fatigue, and weakness were relieved or eliminated in patients troubled by these symptoms, whereas the herb produced a calming effect on emotionally excited patients.

Nervous Tension. Eleuthero extract was tested on telegraph operators. It is known that this type of work requires quick reaction time, deep concentration, physical endurance, and exact coordination of movement. After taking the extract, performance improved. There was finer coordination of mental and physical reflexes, endurance and stamina increased, and the number of mistakes the operators made was significantly reduced.

In other cases radiotelegraph operators were given a daily dose of eleuthero extract for three days. The number of errors decreased, and the operation quality improved.

Diabetes. Professor I. I. Brekhman of the Institute of Biologically Active Substances at Vladivostok reports:

> In patients suffering from light and moderate-gravity diabetes, the use of eleutherococcus extract in a dose of 40 drops three times daily resulted in a reduction of the blood sugar level by 15 to 25mg%. In some cases the positive shifts were still more pronounced. For example, in patient Z (female) who had received a one month course of eleutherococcus treatment, the blood sugar level fell from 140mg%, and the urine sugar decreased gradually from 4 percent first, down to 3, then to 1, and at the end of the treatment down to 0.5 percent. Most patients showed considerable improvement of their general state; weakness and fatigability became less pronounced, thirst and itching troubled them to a much lesser extent.

Eyesight. The effect of eleuthero liquid extract on vision acuity was studied on young subjects with normal vision. One hour after taking the extract, vision enhancement increased from 1.15–1.16 to 1.26–1.32. Eight hours later, vision acuity increased from 1.40 to 1.52 and remained at the enhancement level of 1.25 for 32 hours. Vision returned to normal at the end of the second day.

The extract was also found to enhance color perception in persons with normal vision and in persons who were color blind. In conditions of color blindness, eleuthero extract was given in a dose of 2 milliliters. This provided normal color vision for 36 hours.

Crewmen troubled with a sense of sharp pain in the eyes, photophobia (inability to withstand light), and rapid fatigability while working on a research ship during long-term navigation were given a daily dose of 36 to 40 drops of eleuthero extract for one month. At the end of that time, they no longer complained of their symptoms.

Methods of Using Eleuthero

Eleuthero is generally sold on the market under the more common name of Siberian ginseng. The root is available in the form of fluid extracts, tablets, and as powder contained in capsules. Or the leaves may be obtained and prepared as tea.

A super potent form of Siberian ginseng which grows wild on the remote islands of Japan in an environment free of pollutants and pesticides is also available in the form of capsulated powder. The product is called Enax™. Two to four capsules are taken daily, swallowed with a glass of water before breakfast or between meals. Or the powder may be emptied from the capsules into a cup of warm water, then strained and taken as tea.

As a general course of eleuthero fluid extract, Professor Brekhman recommends 20 to 40 drops in water, before meals, repeated two or three times a day to make a total dose of 80 drops. A treatment course lasts 25 to 30 days. If necessary, repeated courses are taken at one- or two-week intervals.

Note. According to reports in Soviet medical journals, side effects from eleuthero are rare. Occasionally there can be slight drowsiness immediately after taking a dose, in which case it should be taken with meals. If short-term sleeping disturbances are noticed, eleuthero should not be taken directly before bedtime. Eleuthero is also reported to be relatively contraindicated for extreme forms of high blood pressure, severe menstrual bleeding, excessively rapid heart beat, and irregular heart rhythm (commonly referred to as skipped beats).

GARLIC

Botanical Name: *Allium sativum*
Common Names: Clove Garlic, Poor Man's Treacle

Garlic is a member of the lily family along with onions, shallots, and leeks. It is a perennial and one of the most common of the flavoring herbs.

Early Medicinal Uses

The remedial use of garlic is age-old. For thousands of years it has been used to treat many diseases that are being studied today in modern laboratories. The Roman historian Pliny the Elder stated that garlic had "very powerful properties" which could cure over 60 different ailments, and claimed that even its odor would drive away scorpions and serpents. The Greek dramatist Aristophanes regarded the juice of garlic as a restorer of masculine vigor. Hippocrates used the herb to treat a variety of health problems including wounds, skin disorders, and tumors.

In the second century, Dioscorides, a Greek medic who accompanied the Roman armies as their official physician, specified garlic for all lung and intestinal disorders occurring among the soldiers. He also claimed that "garlic doth cleareth the arteries." Garlic was known, too, in China from the earliest times and was cited in the *Calendar of Hsia*, a book written 2,000 years before the birth of Christ.

Modern Remedial Uses Of Garlic

Garlic is classed as antiseptic, antiviral, antibacterial, anti-inflammatory, antifungal, expectorant, diuretic, diaphoretic, and vermifuge. Its constituents include iron, copper, manganese, calcium, zinc, potassium, magnesium, 33 sulfur compounds, 17 amino acids, and vitamins A, B_1, and C.

Garlic is also one of the richest plant sources of germanium, a mineral which strengthens the immune system. The *Allergy Research Review* states:[5]

> The inability of modern medical science to deal effectively with the AIDS epidemic has focused attention on human vulnerability to viral disease in general, especially in a setting of immune imbalance. It is often the body's own interferon response to viral exposure that determines the course of infection. Organic germanium is a potent stimulus to interferon production, which accounts at least in part for its well-established antiviral activity. Although germanium is not currently being widely used by AIDS patients, it was strongly recommended for clinical testing by Dr. Kaneo Yamada, the director of AIDS Research for the Japanese Ministry of Health and Welfare.

Selenium, another essential nutrient richly provided by garlic, is an excellent antioxidant and overall immune enhancer.

Doctors Lidia Kiremedjian-Schumacher and G. Stotsky, authors of a review of studies[6] concerned with immune response noted that "a deficiency of selenium appears to result in immunosuppression, whereas supplementation with low doses of selenium appear to result in augmentation and/or restoration of immunologic functions."

Garlic: Nature's Healer

Garlic has undergone numerous scientific studies to determine its healing aspects. Ailments such as intestinal disorders, high blood pressure, respiratory infections, athlete's foot, infections of the eyes and ears, inflammation or infection of the vagina, lip and mouth disease, acne, arthritis, and lumbago have responded favorably to garlic therapy.

Studies have also demonstrated that garlic attacks more than 23 types of bacteria as well as 70 types of fungi and yeast including *Candida albicans.* Many experiments in the U.S., Japan, and other countries have shown that adequate amounts of garlic in the diet may protect against some forms of cancer. For example, tests on lab animals were conducted by Dr.. Michael Wargovich[7], a biologist at Houston's Anderson Hospital and Tumor Institute. Mice were fed a garlic compound before exposing them to a potent carcinogen which causes cancer of the colon. These mice developed 75% fewer tumors than other mice used in the same study who were not fed garlic. In a further study in which mice were exposed to a carcinogen that affects the esophagus, not one of the garlic-treated mice developed cancer.

Garlic Protects Against Cancer

In China, a study reported[8] some years ago indicated that garlic offers protection against some human cancers. In the province of Ganshan, the rate of stomach cancer was only 3.5 per 100,000 among the residents who regularly ate 20 grams of garlic each day. However, in nearby Quixia, the people rarely eat garlic and the death rate from the same type of cancer was 40 per 100,000. Researchers found that garlic reduced the concentrations on nitrites (precursors which can cause cancer) in the gastric juices of Ganshan residents, thereby offering protection against the formation of stomach cancer.

Other Cancer Studies

Dr. Gerbhard Schauzer, a biochemist at the University of California in San Diego, explains that garlic helps prevent cancer through the action of its constituents, especially selenium, which he refers to as a "cancer fighting agent." He and his colleagues conducted extensive studies of the relationship between cancer deaths and the dietary intake of selenium. Various types of cancers such as tumors of the breast, colon, prostate, ovary, and lung were included in the study. These researchers found that there were fewer cancer death rates where selenium intake was high. Dr. Schauzer believes that if every woman in America began taking selenium supplements today or followed a diet high in selenium, the breast cancer rate in this country would decline drastically in a few years.[9]

Dr. Schaumberger, a cancer researcher of Cleveland, also found that the higher the blood levels of selenium, the lower the incidence of cancer. He advises people to increase their intake of selenium to 200 micrograms per day, because "it can reduce the cancer rate dramatically for some types of cancer, particularly cancer of the colon, breast, esophagus, tongue, stomach, intestines, rectum, and bladder."[10]

Dr. D. Frost, former researcher at Dartmouth Medical School's Trace Element Laboratory, states: "There is damn good evidence that selenium has anti-cancer value. If we want to avoid getting cancer we should be sure to get enough selenium."[11]

People are advised to stay within the range of 200 to 300 micrograms of selenium per day, as toxicity can occur with prolonged use of highly excessive amounts such as 2,400 tp 3,000 micrograms per day. It is important when buying selenium tablets to check the label to make certain that selenium is combined with yeast, as this combination has been found to be more effective.

Food Sources of Selenium

Along with garlic, other examples of foods which contain selenium include seafood, chicken, lamb, whole wheat bread, whole grain cereals, and organ meats such as liver and kidney. In addition, data taken from studies at the Wakunaga Research Center of Japan have shown that a special garlic extract called Kyolic® contains up to seven times more of the herb's essential nutrients, including selenium and germanium, than any other garlic product.

Garlic and AIDS

The most common fungal infection of adult patients with AIDS in the U.S. is candidiasis (white patches of yeast ulcers in the mouth, throat, and esophagus). A patient with these symptoms visited the office of Dr. Tariq Abdullah, director of the AK Bar Clinic of Panama City, Florida. Instead of following the usual medical procedure of treating the patient with antifungal medications, Dr. Abdullah prescribed a special preparation of garlic instead. In two weeks the infection was gone, and Dr. Abdullah said the patient felt 1,000% better.

The potential of garlic as a treatment of AIDS was discussed at the Fifth International AIDS Conference in Montreal.[12] Abdullah presented impressive findings from a 12-week study which showed that seven AIDS patients in Jacksonville and New Orleans improved after taking the special garlic extract. "You can't take seven of anything and say it's certain that this is what's going on," said Abdullah, but results are "suggestive that garlic can play a very helpful role in the treatment of AIDS patients and more studies are justified."

Initially there were 10 patients in the study, but three could not comply with the regimen and died. The seven who participated were given an aged processed garlic liquid extract called Kyolic® Special Garlic Preparation (SPG), manufactured by Wakunaga Pharmaceutical Company of Japan. For the first six weeks, patients took 10 capsules of the garlic extract daily, and the amount was increased to 20 capsules for the last six weeks. By the end of the test study, all seven patients showed a 3- to 14-fold increase in the activity of key immune cells.

Abdullah reported that three of the patients who had sores and two patients with diarrhea no longer had these symptoms by the end of the test. In two patients with genital herpes, symptoms ceased.

The Florida medical team believes that some of the valuable constituents in garlic may be lost if the cloves are cooked, so they chose the Kyolic® garlic product instead, a preparation that is not processed with heat. They report, "Cold-aged whole clove garlic preparations offer the greatest medicinal value, possibly including prevention and therapy for AIDS patients."[13]

A Further Word about Kyolic®

When fresh clove garlic is cut or crushed, a sulfur compound known as allinin is converted to allicin, a harsh irritant which some people cannot tolerate, as it may cause irritation of the mouth and esophagus or further irritate such conditions as stomach ulcers. To correct this problem, Dr. Eugene Schnell, a chemist who had spent years studying Oriental herb remedies in Japan, joined forces with Manji Wakunaga, a strong advocate of herbal medicine. They discovered that through a 20-month cold-aging process of whole garlic, allinin is converted to allicin, which is then converted to more beneficial compounds free of irritation and odor.

In the U.S. this naturally cold-aged preparation is called Kyolic®; in Japan Kyoleopin™; and in Canada Leopin™.

Kyolic® is listed in the *Physicians Desk Reference for Non-Prescription Drugs*[14], a book used by 300,000 medical practitioners in the United States.

Various Forms of Kyolic® Garlic

Kyolic® garlic is grown in healthy, mineral-rich soil, in virgin woodlands free of pesticides and inorganic fertilizers. After undergoing the 20-month cold-aging process, it passes through 250 quality control tests before packaging. It is available on the market in various forms; for example, as powder contained in capsules, as bottled liquid extract with a container of empty gelatin capsules, and in liquid only. The empty capsules are easily filled with the use of the handy spouted bottle and taken immediately. If left to stand, the capsules quickly dissolve.

Kyolic® is also available in combination with other nutritive substances such as garlic/lecithin, garlic/vitamin C, and garlic/parsley/alfalfa.

Directions for using any of these Kyolic® garlic products are given on the labels of the bottles.

Case Studies Show Health Benefits of Kyolic® Garlic

"Jud's allergies are worse in the summer months: hay fever symptoms, he's tired, very short tempered, and irritable.

"The past three winters have been full of earaches, sore throats, strep infections, colds, and flu bugs. It seemed if he played outside in the wind or cold, within one or two days he had something wrong. If someone at the school or church had something, he had caught it within the following week. We were desperate; every two or three weeks poor Jud was at the doctor's office getting a shot or medicine for something.

"In March, our pediatrician told us that Jud's tonsils would have to be removed. He was having a great deal of trouble breathing and swallowing. That was the last shot of penicillin and the last bottle of antibiotic we've given Jud. When the antibiotic was finished, we began giving him three Kyolic® tablets per day.

"We have seen a big change in Jud. His appearance is healthy. He had lost some weight even though he was growing taller. He's gained 10 pounds, still thin but filling out. His face is pink and there are no black circles under his eyes anymore. He also used to scratch his arms and legs; it looked like eczema. We didn't know for sure, but we no longer use the itch medicine or the antibiotic stuff in a tube. He just doesn't itch anymore.

"Jud sleeps better and longer now. There is no more itching and scratching. The running nose, swollen eyes are better. After actually cutting the grass he has some redness, but it's bearable. The swollen tonsils have gone down and Jud's energy level is up! He plays ball and he's outside at all hours now and he doesn't get sick. In February, Jud had the sniffles for a few days. All we gave him besides the Kyolic® were tissues." —Mrs. Y. J.

"I started taking Kyolic® liquid garlic (plain), approximately 2 to 4 capsules per day. I work at a car manufacturing plant and had happened to be working on the line at the time I first started taking the garlic product. I was continually tired and would come home every night exhausted. All I wanted to do was lie on the couch. However, after taking the garlic I found that I had more energy. In addition, I lost about 10 pounds, and my high blood pressure is totally under control. In the past, I had taken medicine for this condition on occasion.

"My wife started taking Kyolic® garlic after she noticed the improvement in my energy. She also experienced a noticeable increase in energy, lost weight, and just generally feels better. Both of us cannot go more than a week without our garlic. We have also been taking two capsules of powdered Kyolic® garlic every day. My wife also says the garlic is great for her acne problem—she doesn't use antibiotics anymore."—M. W.

"I have an experience for you. Early this year when I was on the West Coast, I saw a lady with a severe yeast problem—almost unable to eat anything, a lot of gas, bloating, discomfort, poor digestion, etc. She had tried everything including Nystatin, with minimal help. We told her to take liquid Kyolic®, 3 teaspoonfuls three times a day, along with a special diet, and some other suggestions. She called me three months later to say that within two weeks her symptoms were all gone. She also told me she had hypercholesterolemia, with it usually running around 350 in spite of being a total vegetarian. With the use of a lot of oat bran and charcoal, she had been able to get it down to 305. But at the end of two months on Kyolic®, she had the cholesterol checked again for interest and it had dropped to 220! She said it has not been that low in her adult life (she is now 45 years old."—C. E., MD.

MINOR BUPLEURUM COMBINATION

This is a traditional Chinese formula consisting of the following herbs: bupleurum, panax ginseng, ginger, licorice, pinellia, scute, and jujube. These herbs produce the following immune strengthening effects according to Oriental research studies:

- Bupleurum stimulates antibody and interferon production.
- Panax ginseng is an adaptogen. Due to the herb's antioxidant components, it can slow the aging process caused

by free radicals. The herb also contains polysaccharides, which strengthen the immune system's defense against invading antigens.

- Ginger stimulates phagocytic activity against toxic substances and infections.
- Licorice is antiviral and antiatherosclerotic.
- Pinellia induces production of interferon, which can fight viral and other infections.
- Scute and jujube have demonstrated antiallergic effects.

Minor bupleurum combination has become immensely popular among the people of Japan during the last decade. The elderly use it as a tonic to boost their declining immunity, while the young use it to help improve their resistance to disease. It is frequently used to prevent the common cold and is recommended to assist recovery during periods of illness. (This product is also available on the U.S. market in capsulated form.)

Minor bupleurum combination and other Chinese herbal formulas are being used in Japan for the treatment of AIDS, and the results have reportedly been encouraging.[15]

OTHER IMMUNE BOOSTING HERBS

A number of other herbs have been receiving good reports as strengtheners of the immune system. Among the most prominent of these are chaparral, Pau d'Arco, tang-kuei, hoelen, various Chinese herbal formulas, and the Suma™ brand of *Pfaffia paniculata*.

SUMMARY

1. The health of the immune system depends on the harmonious interaction of all the components which permit the body to recognize the presence of disease microorganisms and to reject or destroy them.
2. Imbalances or a severe disruption of the immune function can result in a vast number of illnesses.
3. Evidence shows that the use of certain herbs, along with correct eating habits, exercise, adequate sleep, and other health practices can strengthen the immune system.
4. Echinace contains compounds that are antiviral and antibacterial as well as immunostimulating properties.
5. Astragalus is highly acclaimed as probably the most important of all the deep immune tonics, supporting immune strength at a very deep level.

6. A combination of immune boosting herbs according to Chinese traditional principles is known as Astragalus Eight Herbs Formula.

7. Reishi and shiitake mushrooms bolster immunity and stimulate health.

8. Eleuthero, popularly called Siberian ginseng, ranks as "King of the Adaptogens."

9. Garlic is a rich source of selenium and germanium, essential nutrients which are excellent antioxidants and overall immune enhancers.

10. Kyolic®, a special cold-aged garlic preparation, contains up to seven times more of the bulb's important constituents, including selenium and germanium, than any other garlic product.

11. Minor bupleurum combination produces immune strengthening effects.

ENDNOTES

1. *The Nature Doctor* (Teufen AR Switzerland: Bioforce-Verlag).

2. *Nonspecific Enhancement of Intrinsic Resistance to Infection by Echinacin* K. Ch. Schimmel and G. T. Werner (Ther. d. Gegnw., 1981).

3. "Editorial," *Medical Tribune*, March 28, 1984.

4. *Hokubei Mainichi*, October 24, 1980.

5. Fall 1987.

6. *Environmental Research*, No. 42, 1987.

7. "New Dietary Anticarcinogens and Prevention of Gastrointestinal Cancer." *Dis. Col. Rectum*, Jan. 31, 1988.

8. X. Mei et al., "Garlic and Gastric Cancer." *Acta Nutr. Sinica*, Vol. 4, p. 53, 1982.

9. E. Mishara, *National Enquirer*, June 14, 1978.

10. Ibid.

11. Ibid.

12. June 4–9, 1989.

13. T. H. Abdullah, O. Kandil, A. Elkadi, and J. Carter, "Garlic Revisited: Therapeutics for the Major Diseases of Our Times?" *J. Nat'l Med. Assn.*, 1988.

14. 1984.

15. Pi-Kwang Sung, Ph.D., *OHAI NEWSLETTER*, Winter 1987.

CHAPTER 2

LIVER AND GALLBLADDER PROBLEMS

Writing for the *Los Angeles Times*[1], Thelma K. Thiel stated: "Most Americans think cirrhosis of the liver is a disease of alcoholics and hepatitis is a disease of drug addicts. Not true! Even babies die of cirrhosis and half of the hepatitis cases are among children and teenagers."

An estimated 30 million people in the U.S. suffer from liver-related disorders, and these diseases are the third leading cause of death in the nation. Lost work time and medical costs for liver problems exceed 14 billion dollars annually.

What Your Liver Does for You

Your liver has a host of duties to perform to keep you in good health. Here is a partial list: It makes antibodies to help protect you from infectious diseases; aids your digestive process by manufacturing bile; regulates blood clotting to keep you from bleeding to death from a cut; stores various minerals, vitamins, and sugars to prevent shortages in your physical energy; controls the production and excretion of cholesterol; regulates fats, carbohydrates, and protein processing.

The liver is also a marvelous built-in toxic waste disposal unit which filters out an incredible number of chemical impurities in the blood by transforming toxins into metabolites capable of being excreted.

The Liver Under Siege

For thousands of years the existing environment was a natural one in all essentials. But around the middle of the last

23

century, humans began to develop an increasing number of substances that did not exist in nature, and this practice has expanded at a frightening rate. Today we are exposed to a multitude of toxins in our air, water, food, clothing, and homes, and the result has been a wide spectrum of illnesses including liver damage.

Toxic matter is released into the atmosphere from automobile exhaust pipes, factories, crop dusters, jet airplanes, and huge manufacturing plants. Air pollution is eating away at marble-surfaced buildings and killing fish in lakes in the wild. Sometimes industries are forced to close when air pollution becomes trapped by weather inversion.

Numerous home owners spray toxic pesticides on their lawns, trees, and bushes, or hire professionals to do the job. Advertisers encourage us to spray for pests around the home by using spray cans or pest strips. Other exposures to indoor chemical pollution include room fresheners, disinfectant sprays, dry cleaning materials, paints, varnishes, tobacco smoke, newsprint, detergents, and bleaching agents. Even our clothing is made of blends of synthetics, or the material has been chemically treated for permanent press or fumigated with formaldehyde.

In addition it is almost impossible to buy food in a supermarket that has not been processed in some way by chemical additives, preservatives, flavorings, and colorings. The National Academy of Science has stated that pesticides on food cause about 20,000 cases of cancer a year. Our food contains varieties of 2,700 FDA approved additives. Nitrates and nitrites are commonly used in bacon, smoked fish, canned ham, sausage, and many pressed meats. It has been demonstrated that nitrites can combine with substances known as amines, and this action can create new compounds which are cancer-causing agents. Seafood has frequently become contaminated by mercury, resulting in serious diseases and death. Even fruits and vegetables contain their share of toxic pesticides.

Such list of contaminants to which we are exposed could go on and on. This state of affairs has caused some medical authorities to state that *all* of us suffer from some type of liver impairment to a greater or lesser degree.

The Liver Needs Help

The liver is a powerful defender against toxic pollutants. It can tolerate a certain amount of contamination, but if it is overloaded it becomes damaged or diseased. Some of the symptoms which can indicated dysfunction of this vital organ may include "liverish" migraine headache, stomach distress, excess gas, visual disturbances, nausea, constipation, diarrhea, dark-colored urine (which contains bile), white or greyish stools, nervousness, depression, anxiety, and insomnia. Severe impairment of the liver can progress to hepatitis, jaundice, gallstones, cirrhosis, and cancer of the liver. Toxic overload also weakens the immune system, lowering resistance to mental and physical illnesses.

A Word about the Gallbladder

The gallbladder is a pear-shaped muscular sack which stores and concentrates bile secreted by the liver into the small intestine. The bile helps to absorb and emulsify fats. As soon as food reaches the duodenum from the stomach, a nervous reflex causes the common bile closure duct to open and the stored bile is then released. The bile saturates the food and activates the pancreatic juices that have entered at the same time, causing further digestion of the food to take place. The more fat the food contains, the greater the amount of bile that is released.

Dr. Alfred Vogel of Switzerland[2] explains that the stimulus which causes the common bile duct closure to open and the gallbladder to contract so that just the right amount of bile is released into the duodenum must obviously depend on a delicately balanced nerve mechanism. If this mechanism is thrown out of gear, "spasms are then set up and organs become cramped and contracted and the gall is forced back into the liver or even bloodstream when we shall have a jaundice on our hands." In the condition of jaundice, the skin and the whites of the eyes become yellowish.

Gallstones

An excess of fatty rich foods in the diet can injure the gallbladder and increase the chances of forming gallstones. These stones can range in size from tiny gravel to that of a small plum. They may consist of different substances, but those formed of cholesterol are the most common. (Herbalists report that cholesterol-type stones have the greatest possibility of being dissolved.)

Sometimes a gallstone is pushed out of the bladder by a flood of gall and becomes lodged in the common bile duct. This causes extreme pain known as gallstone colic and is frequently accompanied by nausea, vomiting, chills, and sweating. In severe cases there may be symptoms of cardiac irregularity. If the bile is blocked because of the stones and cannot leave the gallbladder, it returns to the liver and enters the bloodstream.

Medics point out that a gallbladder attack does not occur without some indications of gallbladder disease having existed for some time. The diet had probably consisted of rich, fatty foods which eventually become indigestible, resulting in stomach distress, heartburn, gas, and belching. The time comes when suddenly an attack occurs that produces a sharp pain in the region of the lower ribs on the right side and radiates to the right shoulder, although it may go through to the back. The cramp-like pain can be very intense, causing the person to double up in an attempt to relieve the agony. Vomiting can also occur during the attack.

HERB REMEDIES FOR LIVER AND GALLBLADDER PROBLEMS

In addition to using any kind of the following herbal aids for the liver and gallbladder, the diet should consist of foods which support the work of these important organs. Generally, meals should be small and frequent, low in fat, and rich in fresh vegetables, especially artichokes, dandelion greens, red beets, cucumbers, swiss chard, and beet greens. Lowfat yogurt and dandelion coffee are also beneficial. Overly refined foods, sugars, fried foods, artificial sweeteners, beverages containing caffeine, and foods contaminated by chemical colorings, flavorings, and preservatives should be avoided.

Various supplements are also important to the health of the liver and gallbladder. Among these are vitamins A, C, and the B complex, plus minerals and amino acids.

MILK THISTLE

Botanical Name: *Silybum marianum*
Common Names: Our Lady's Thistle, Marian Thistle

This tall plant of green prickly leaves marked with white veins is found growing on hedge banks, roadsides, farms, and pastures. The bright purple flowering heads at the end of the stalks appear from June to August.

There is a legend that the white markings on the leaves originated from the milk of the Virgin Mary that once fell upon the plant; therefore it was called Our Lady's Thistle, and the Latin name has the same derivation.

A Timeless Remedy

In 1597 Gerard, a prominent early herbalist, wrote: "My opinion is that this (milk thistle) is the best remedy that grows against all melancholy diseases." The word *melancholy* is taken from the Greek, "black bile," and in Gerard's day referred to any liver or biliary derangement. Culpepper, 1646 A.D., often referred to as the Father of English Herbology, recommended an infusion of the roots and seeds of milk thistle as a treatment for jaundice and for breaking and expelling stones. Writing in 1694, Westmacott says of the plant, "It is a friend to the liver and blood."

Early in the twentieth century, the Eclectics[3] used the herb for treating various ailments including liver congestion. Around the same time, family physicians employed preparations of milk thistle in their practices. Dr. Liebach reported cases of jaundice and enlargement of the liver which were cured with its use. From 10 to 15 drops of the tincture were taken in a little water three times a day.

In more recent years, Dr. Eric Powell wrote that milk thistle has a specific action on the liver and that indications for its use are "when the liver is sore, when the patient is subject to 'liverishness' and jaundice." He said that even serious liver disorders have been known to respond to the herb when other remedies have failed.

Scientific Research on Milk Thistle

Milk thistle has attracted considerable scientific interest, especially in Europe where commercial preparations of the herb are being hailed as superb liver tonics and are also used to treat severe liver disorders such as cirrhosis and hepatitis.

Silymarin, the active constituent of milk thistle, was first isolated back in the late 1960s. The main active compounds of silymarin are silybin, silychristin, and silydianin. Researchers learned of its value for liver problems when Dr. G. Vogel of Germany conducted a study using the herbal extract for treating 60 patients suffering from amanita death cap mushroom poisoning, which attacks and destroys the liver. Dr. Vogel reported that results ranged from "amazing to spectacular." Whereas the death rate using modern supportive measures is usually 30% to 40%, all 60 patients taking the milk thistle extract lived.

Clinical Studies Continue

Since that time, clinical studies with milk thistle extract have been conducted on more that 2,000 patients and numerous lab animal suffering from some type of liver dysfunction. All reportedly experienced marked health benefits. These and continued studies have shown that the herbal extract regenerates the liver cells. Studies have also shown that ailments such as cirrhosis, hepatitis, and other liver diseases are prevented and in many cases reversed and cured by its use. In addition, the extract protects the liver against the onslaught of toxic chemical pollutants, alcohol, and various drug medications, and without any side effects.

Dr. G. Vogel reports[4]:

> Dr. Gerok of Freiburg, Germany, who chaired the symposium *Flavonoids and the Liver*, stated in his conclusions that the therapeutic value of silymarin for the treatment of toxic metabolic liver damage was established beyond all doubt. In addition, a recent multi-center double blind study proved without any doubt that the survival period of cirrhotic patients was significantly prolonged by silymarin.

Dr. V. Fintelman, in his report *Toxic-Metabolic Hepatic Dysfunction and Its Management*,[5] stated that for proper treatment of the liver it is ideal to avoid the causes which can damage this vital organ, but that is not always possible. Therefore, it is important to know that milk thistle extract "will reliably reverse toxic hepatic dysfunction of different origins" such as alcohol, drug, and chemical induced toxicity.

In Germany, commercial preparations of milk thistle extract are being manufactured for serious liver ailments such as cirrhosis and hepatitis as well as tonics for protection, regeneration, and strengthening of the liver. These extracts are selling at the rate of almost 200 million dollars annually.

Method of Using Milk Thistle

There are a number of extracts on the market which contain silymarin, the active ingredient of milk thistle seeds. Many also contain conutrients to help the liver do its job and to regenerate itself when it has been damaged by toxins. Check with your health food store or herb firm for the variety of milk thistle products available. Instructions on how the product is to be taken, plus the list of ingredients it contains, are cited on the labels.

FRINGE TREE

Botanical Name: *Chionanthus virginica*
Common Names: American Fringe Tree, Snow Flowers, Old Man's Beard, White Fringe

This large shrub or small tree is indigenous to the U.S. and grows wild on river banks, thickets, and bluffs. Because of the charming appearance of its fragrant snow-white flowers and green glossy foliage, it is cultivated as an ornamental plant in gardens and parks. The common name, fringe tree, is derived from the fringe-like petals of the flowers.

Early Uses of Fringe Tree

Fringe tree was a popular remedy among the American Indians. The Choctaws boiled the root bark and used the decoction to bathe wounds and skin irritations, while the pulped bark was applied as a wet poultice for painful bruises and severe lacerations. Some tribes drank decoctions to relieve biliousness, bilious sick headaches, sore throat, and sore mouth. The early colonists learned of the Indian herbal remedy and used it for intermittent fevers of a bilious character and for "liverish" headaches.

Fringe Tree from Past to Present

For a long time, medical doctors rejected Indian herbalism as the superstitious nonsense of an uncivilized people. But gradually, as the centuries passed, a number of native folk remedies came to the attention of some physicians, who found that many were of great value.

Around the turn of the century, Professor I. J. M. Goss gave an impressive account in which he credited the use of fringe tree with curing him of a severe case of jaundice after orthodox treatments by several of the best physicians had failed to help. At the time of his illness he was still in medical school. Accepting the suggestion of a fellow student that he try a folk remedy of fringe tree, he prepared a tincture of the root bark in gin and took a tablespoonful before each meal. He reported:

> In a few days my appetite began to improve, and my skin very rapidly cleared, and in some ten days my jaundice was gone; my skin was clear of bilious hue, and I felt like another man. I subsequently met with many cases of jaundice, and found the remedy so prompt to remove it that I published my experience in the *Eclectic Medical Journal of Philadelphia*, since which time I have used it in a great many cases with success. I now use a saturated tincture . . . Dose: 1 drachm (approx. 1 teaspoon) 3 times a day.

Around the same time, Dr. J. A. Henning also found the herb remedy to be effective for the same condition. He wrote:

In functional jaundice, fringe tree is nearly a specific, given in doses of a fluid extract of from fifteen to twenty drops in a small glass of water every three to six hours as may be indicated in the case.

Later Reports

Over the years that followed, a number of doctors and medical journals began reporting on the remedial value of fringe tree. Consider the following examples:

- Dr. Felter of Lloyd's reported that fringe tree is one of the most effective remedies employed in cases of gallstones, jaundice, bilious colic, and acute or chronic inflammation of the liver.

- Dr. Swinburne Clymer[6] cited fringe tree as "the liver remedy *par excellence*, when there is tenderness over the region of the liver, in jaundice and gallstones, bilious colic, acute dyspepsia, acute and chronic inflammation of the liver and in biliousness of alcoholism." He gave the dosage as five to ten drops of the tincture in water, before meals.

- *Potter's New Cyclopaedia of Botanical Drugs and Preparations*[7] lists the remedial action of fringe tree as "prompt and efficacious in liver derangements and also in jaundice and gallstones." The recommended dosage of the liquid extract is cited as 5 to 30 drops in water.

- Dr. Jon Evans[8] of England recommended the fluid extract of fringe tree as an aid in expelling gallstones and in preventing their formation. He added that its use is effective in jaundice and liver ailments as well. The dosage he advised is 12 drops of the extract in a little water three times daily before meals.

TUMERIC

Botanical Name: *Curcuma longa*
Common Name: Curcuma

Tumeric is native to Southern Asia and is cultivated in China, Java, and Bengal. It is a perennial plant with oblong roots or tubers deep orange or reddish-brown inside and yellowish externally. When dried, cuttings from the roots produce a yellow powder which has a peculiar fragrant odor and bitterish taste.

Commercially, tumeric is employed in the manufacture of curry powders and is sometimes used as a coloring agent.

Medicinal Uses

Since earliest times tumeric has been accepted as a remedy for liver ailments. It was first listed in the ancient Chinese text *Tang Pen Tsao* (A.D. 659) under the common name of curcuma. In Chinese medicine the plant is used for various ailments including gallstones and jaundice.

Recently, scientific studies have demonstrated that curcumin, the yellow pigment of tumeric, has similar liver-protecting effects to that of silymarin (milk thistle).[9] It is one of the ingredients of various liver tonics sold in health food stores.

DANDELION

Botanical Name: *Leontodon taraxacum*
Common Names: Lion's Tooth, Priest's Crown, Puffball

Dandelion is a common plant native to Greece but has spread to almost every part of the world. The purplish flower stalks which rise from the root are hollow and smooth and bear single heads of light golden yellow flowers.

The name *taraxacum* is derived from the Greek *taraxos* (disorder) and *akos* (remedy) indicating the plant's value as a healing agent.

Dandelion: Friend of the Liver

Dandelion root contains inulin, potash, pectin, sugar, levulin, and a good amount of alkaline salts. Due to its content of potash, it is considered an effective diuretic. The root also contains two alkaloids, the most valuable of which is taraxacin. According to Dr. Bartram (Fellow of the National Institute of Medical Herbalists, and Fellow of the Royal Society of Herbalists, England), "Hepatitis or inflammation of the liver, and jaundice when uncomplicated readily yield to the taraxacin of dandelion."

Dandelion greens contain 7,000 units of vitamin A per ounce and provide an abundance of vitamins B_1 and C, along with cholin, a factor of the B complex which science has found be essential to proper liver function.

Dandelion is used to promote the formation of bile, to stimulate the liver to detoxify poisons, and to remove excess water from the system in conditions of edema resulting from liver ailments. It is also said to be effective in the treatment of jaundice and hepatitis.

Methods of Using Dandelion

Decoction: One ounce of dandelion roots is simmered slowly in 1-1/2 pints of water for 10 minutes. It is then strained, and one cup is taken an hour after meals three times a day.

Fluid Extract: If a fluid extract is used, 1/2 teaspoon is taken in a wine glass of water after meals three times daily.

Dandelion Greens: The greens are very nutritious and may be boiled and served like spinach, or the fresh young leaves can be used as salads. Herbalists maintain that dandelion salad cleanses, stimulates, and heals the liver and should always be on the table throughout the spring.

Dandelion Coffee: When dandelion coffee is used as a substitute for regular coffee, it reportedly imparts a beneficial effect on the whole system, helping the liver and kidneys do their job. It is also considered excellent for preventing the formation of gallstones in persons susceptible to them.

Note. In earlier times, dandelion coffee was prepared by roasting the dried roots in the oven and then grinding them for use. Today, however, dandelion coffee has become a commercial product and is available on the market. It is a natural beverage and does not contain caffeine.

Homeopathic Formula

William Boericke, M.D., cited the following characteristics and guiding symptoms for the use of dandelion according to homeopathy (the patient may suffer from any number of the symptoms in any one of the groups listed, but not necessarily from all of them).

Taraxacum (Dandelion)

For gastric headaches, bilious attacks with characteristically mapped tongue and jaundiced skin. Flatulence. Hysterical tympanites (distentions of the abdomen due to excess gas in the intestines).

Head—Sensation of great heat on top of head. Sternomastoid muscle very painful to touch.

Mouth—Mapped tongue. Tongue coated with white film, feels raw; comes off in patches, leaving red, sensitive spots. Loss of appetite. Bitter taste and eructions. Salivation.

Abdomen—Liver enlarged and indurated. Sharp stitches in left side. Sensation of bubbles bursting in bowels. Tympanites. Evacuation difficult.

Extremities—Very restless limbs. Neuralgia of knee; better pressure. Limbs painful to touch.

Fever—Chilliness after eating, worse drinking; fingertips cold.

Bitter taste—Heat without thirst, in face, in toes. Sweat on falling asleep.

Skin—Profuse night sweats.

Modalities—Worse resting, lying down, sitting. Better, touch.

Dose: Tincture, to third potency. (Directions are given on the bottle.)

Case Studies

Many people have reported good results with the use of dandelion as a home remedy for liver problems. Following are two of many examples:

"While asking a retired pharmacist if he remembered how a mustard plaster was prepared, I mentioned that a cousin of mine had hepatitis and was not doing very well with the doctor's medication he had been taking for such a long time. The pharmacist told me that dandelion tea was an accepted remedy back in the old days and that many people swore by it. I related this information to my cousin along with the directions the pharmacist gave me for making the decoction. My cousin drank strong cups of it every day and in two months he was cured. I do not know if the remedy would help everyone, but it surely is worth a try." —Mr. R. W.

"I have something I would like to share with you. A few years ago, I and three of my friends came down with hepatitis after returning from an extended trip abroad. As I am a firm believer in natural remedies, I prepared a decoction of dandelion root and drank three to four cups a day for three weeks. At the end of that time I was completely well. My friends who had taken prescription drugs experienced side effects and did not fully recover." —Mrs. M. C.

ARTICHOKE

Botanical Name: *Cynara scolymus*
Common Names: Globe Artichoke, Garden Artichoke

The artichoke is the world's oldest cultivated food plant and was grown by the early Romans and Greeks. It was introduced into England in the sixteenth century both as a food and as an ornamental plant in monastery gardens.

The flower stems of the artichoke grow erect, and each are terminated by a large globular head of spiny scales, greenish-purple in color. These envelop a mass of blue flowers in the center. In an immature state, the flower heads contain parts that are edible.

Remedial Uses

The artichoke is classed as a cholagogue and has a long-standing reputation in treating many liver ailments. Dr. Alfred Vogel writes:[10]

> Again and again I am surprised to what extent arti-chokes help in the case of liver-disorders. A period of only 2–3 days is quite sufficient to furnish convincing proof of their efficacy as a liver remedy if they are eaten raw, and apart from the carrot, we may therefor count them as one of the most curative dietetic articles we have at our disposal. Raw artichokes are eaten in exactly the same way as cooked ones; one leaf after the other is peeled off to get at their tender part and the inside or the 'hearts' of the artichoke . . . The heart is very tender too, and is as beneficial as the rest of the plant. If cooked artichokes are preferred to the raw ones, they should at least be alternated, because the raw ones have much greater healing power. They should appear at least twice or thrice on the table, and if we want to exploit them fully, we shall want to serve this valuable vegetable daily.

Scientific Evaluation

Scientific evidence supports the use of the artichoke as a liver remedy. Cynarin is the active ingredient contained in the plant, and its highest concentration is in the leaves. According to reports, cynara (artichoke leaves) extract has demonstrated significant liver regenerating and protecting effects. It also stimulates the flow of the bile from the liver to the gallbladder, which makes it useful in the treatment of hepatitis, liver congestion, and other liver problems. Cynara extracts have also been shown to lower cholesterol levels.

CELANDINE

Botanical Name: *Chelidonium majus*
Common Names: Greater Celandine, Tatterwort, Common Celandine

Celandine is a pale green perennial herb indigenous to Europe and naturalized in the U.S. It grows in rich, damp soil along fences, byroads, and waste places. The bright yellow flowers blossom throughout the summer and are arranged at the ends of the stems in loose umbrels.

The name *celandine* comes from the Greek *Chelidon*, "swallow," and was given because the plant is usually in bloom when swallows return to the shores. As early as Culpeper's time (17th century), the herb was used for treating yellow-jaundice, biliary colic, and gallstones.

Reported Uses of Celandine

- Herbalist M. Grieve states that 8 to 10 drops of celandine tincture taken three times a day in water is considered excellent for overcoming sluggish conditions of the liver.
- Dr. Jon Evans reports:[11] "I have used this superlative plant (celandine) for the treatment of countless gallbladder conditions with highly satisfactory results . . . Modern research has only now confirmed its therapeutic action." He tells of the time he was invited by the BBC to give a short interview on herbal medicines. One of the plants he mentioned was celandine, and he cited the case of a patient who had been spared of having an operation for the removal of his gallbladder by its use. Dr. Evans was deluged with letters from listeners asking for further information about the remedy. He says the effort of replying "was happily rewarded by those who later wrote to tell me that they, too, had been cured after using the herbal treatment."

Dr. Evans's Instructions for Using Celandine. Dr. Evans suggests the following methods of using celandine:

> When treating gallstones and biliary colic I have found that the preparation in fluid extract produces the most desirable results:

> 10–12 drops Fluid Extract Chelidonium (celandine) three times a day after meals in a little water.

He also mentions that extract of fringe tree can be combined with celandine:

> Equal proportions of both herbal extracts. Dose: One teaspoonful three times a day in water.

Further Instructions. Dr. Evans explains that while treating gallstones and biliary colic, the diet should consist of fresh fruits, green vegetables, and very lean meat if the patient is not a vegetarian. Lowfat cottage cheese can be included. Starches, sweets, and chocolate are to be avoided, and definitely nothing fried, and no eggs or fats. He recommends dandelion coffee in place of regular coffee.

A Different Approach to Using Celandine

For centuries the Chinese have claimed that repeated awakening from sleep at a certain hour is caused by the dysfunction of a specific organ in the body. They refer to this phenomenon as the "organ-clock." Many nurses have known for some time that regular awakening between the hours of 1 A.M. and 3 A.M. is indicative of a distressed liver. According to the Chinese, it is during these hours that the liver is at the height of its activity. Nurses have reportedly noticed that gallstone colic mainly occurs between the hours of 11 P.M. and 1 A.M., which shows that the production of the gall reaches its peak during the organ-time. Therefore, as a therapeutic counterattack against biliary colic, some homeopaths suggest administering chelidonium 2x, or any other specific remedy, between the hours of 11 P.M. and 1 A.M., and for liver distress between 1 A.M. and 3 A.M.

BARBERRY

Botanical Name: *Berberis vulgaris*
Common Names: Jaundice Berry, Pepperidge Bush

Barberry is a deciduous bush that grows among rocks and gravelly soil in Northeastern states and occasionally on rich grounds in the West. It bears clusters of small pale yellow flowers and branches of bright red oblong berries.

The common name of jaundice berry was given to indicate the plant's remedial use, while the term *pepperidge bush* is from "pepon," a pip, and "rouge," red, as descriptive of the scarlet fruit.

Medicinal Uses

The medicinal action of the root bark is classed as hepatic, tonic, and laxative.

Barberry contains berberine, a yellow crystalline bitter substance which promotes the secretion of bile. The root bark is used by herbalists in conditions of bilious migraine headache, jaundice, general debility, gallstones, and functional derangement of the liver. In Russia it is used for biliary colic, gallbladder inflammation, and to stimulate the flow of bile.

Methods of Preparation

Either of the following methods may be used:

Tinctures: Five to 10 drops in a small glass of water three or four times a day.

Extracts: One-half to 1 teaspoon two or three times a day, in water.

Decoctions: One-half to 1 teaspoon of the root bark is boiled in a cup of water for one minute, then removed from the burner and allowed to stand for five minutes. One-half to 1 cup of the strained decoction is taken during the day, a large mouthful at a time.

Combined Formula: Bitter herbs such as barberry and dandelion are often combined and sold commercially in the form of fluid extracts. One such product consists of barberry, golden seal, dandelion, prickly ash, rhubarb, and gentian. It is used as a liver tonic.

SOYBEAN LECITHIN

Lecithin, (pronounced less-i-thin) consists of bland water-soluble granules refined from soybeans. This remarkable food substance reportedly produces a beneficial effect on the liver, gallbladder, brain, cardiovascular system, and many other parts of the body. It breaks down cholesterol into tiny particles and keeps it in suspension, thereby preventing the cholesterol from precipitating out of the bile to form gallstones. By metabolizing fats, it also reduces the chance of liver degeneration.

Lecithin is the richest natural source of the B vitamins inositol and choline. An excess of digested fats may be combatted by choline, and inositol helps to reduce the amount of the dangerous fatty substance of cholesterol. Lab experiments have shown that when rats were given added amounts of all the B-complex vitamins, particularly inositol, their blood cholesterol rate was vastly reduced.

Medical Studies

According to Dr. R. K. Tompkins and his colleagues, gallstones can be prevented when adequate lecithin is added to the diet. At an annual meeting of the Federation of American Societies for Experimental Biology, these investigators reported their conclusions: Since 90% of human gallstones are composed primarily of cholesterol, it is important to maintain cholesterol in solution in the bile to prevent gallstone formation. They reported on recent studies that have indicated that a class of compounds, called phospholipids, are required to prevent cholesterol precipitation from the bile, and that supplementing the diet with commercial lecithin, the main phospholipid contained in bile, enriched the bile and aided its ability to hold cholesterol in solution.

Other studies conducted in the U.S. and the Soviet Union have also shown that when lecithin is taken daily, gallstones are less likely to form.

How Lecithin Is Used

Lecithin is a potent cholesterol chaser and would be a welcome addition to the diet. It is available as granules, bottled oil, and as capsules of the oil. If using the granules, 1 to 2 tablespoons may be stirred in a glass of water or fruit juice and taken twice a day with meals. If liquid lecithin capsules are used instead, 12 of the capsules are equal to approximately 2 tablespoons of the granules. The bottled oil may be used over salads and as cooking oil.

SUMMARY

1. Exposure to a multitude of toxins in the environment (air, water, food, etc.) results in a wide spectrum of illnesses including liver damage.

2. The liver has the task of eliminating impurities from the blood and performs many other important duties as well.

3. The liver can tolerate a certain amount of toxic pollutants, but if this vital organ is overloaded it becomes damaged or diseased. Toxic overload also weakens the immune system.

4. The gallbladder is a small muscular sack which stores and concentrates bile secreted by the liver.

5. An excess of rich, fatty foods in the diet can injure the gallbladder and lead to the formation of gallstones.

6. Gallstones may consist of different substances, but those formed of cholesterol are the most common.

7. When a gallstone slips out of the gallbladder and becomes lodged in the common bile duct, it causes extreme pain known as gallstone colic.

8. There are many herbs and herbal products that may be used for treating various liver and gallbladder problems.

9. A diet which supports the work of the liver and gallbladder should be adopted along with using any of the herbal remedies. Various supplements are also important to the health of the liver and gallbladder.

ENDNOTES

1. 1982.
2. *The Liver* (Teufen AR Switzerland: Bioforce-Verlag, 1962), pp. 87–88.
3. Doctors who practive a system of medicine derived from several different schools of teaching, such as herbalism, homeopathy, and allopathy.
4. "A Peculiarity Among the Flavenoids—Silymarin, A Compound Active on the Liver." Proceedings of the International Bioflavenoid Symposium, Munich, FRG, 1981.
5. *Zeitschrift fur Phytotherapie*, 1986.
6. *Nature's Healing Agents* (Quakertown, PA: The Humanitarian Society Reg.), 1960.
7. R. C. Wren (London: Sir Isaac Pitman & Sons Ltd.,1956, 7th edition).
8. *Health from Herbs*, September-October 1967.
9. Y. Kiso, Y. Suzuki, Watanabe et al., "Anti-hepatoxic Principles of *Curcuma longa* Rhizomes," *Planta Mexico*, 1983.
10. *The Liver* (Teufen AR Switzerland: Bioforce-Verlag), 1962, p. 156.
11. *Health from Herbs*, September-October 1967.

C H A P T E R 3

HERBS FOR COPING WITH PMS, MENSTRUAL PROBLEMS, AND MENOPAUSE

Premenstrual syndrome (PMS) affects millions of women primarily in their thirties and the condition generally worsens with age. One hundred eighty symptoms have been described, the most common of which are irritability, crying jags, mood swings, fluid retention, cramps, fatigue, back pain, depression, headaches, and temporary weight gain. Other common symptoms include low self-esteem, tender breasts, restlessness, insomnia, acne and skin eruptions, anxiety, and abdominal bloating. The symptoms occur during the six to eight days prior to the onset of menstruation and generally improve after menstruation begins.

For many years physicians had considered PMS to be all in the mind, but a growing number of medical researchers have now presented convincing evidence that the condition is a physically based illness attributed to hormonal imbalances resulting in emotional and physical changes.

In order to identify whether the condition is really PMS, David Baron, deputy clinical director of the National Institute of Mental Health, explains that the cycle of symptoms must be consistent for at least two or three months in a row. Dr. Leslie Hartley Gise of Mount Sinai School of Medicine adds that if the symptoms continue throughout the entire month, the condition is not PMS. "With true PMS," she says, "a woman is completely well two or three weeks out of the month."

Dr. Gise points out that while there is no scientific evidence that dietary management helps PMS, balanced meals high in fibre and low in fat are beneficial.

Menstrual Problems

The majority of young women experience some discomfort with their monthly periods at some time. The most common difficulties are described as follows:

Dysmenorrhea. The most frequent and painful occurrence of menstrual trouble is called menstrual colic or dysmenorrhea. About one in 20 women experience pain severe enough to incapacitate them and to interfere with their work, social life, and studies. In *spasmodic* dysmenorrhea the pain and cramping occurs with the onset of the menses, becomes more intense by the passage of blood clots, and is confined to the area of the lower back and pelvis. In *congestive* dysmenorrhea the pain is felt as a dull ache over the lower abdomen, generally for a few days before the monthly period begins. With the onset of menstruation the pain is usually relieved.

Amenorrhea. In primary conditions of amenorrhea, a young woman has not yet experienced menstruation even though she is past the age when menses should have started. In *secondary* cases she may have started menstruation at the average age, then after a while the periods have stopped. In some women suppression of the menses may result from a sudden shock to the system, either physical or emotional, or from some disturbance in their way of life (e.g., leaving home for the first time to attend a university). It may also occur from exposure to cold or dampness or in the course of an illness.

Menorrhagia. This is a condition of profuse menstrual bleeding with each monthly period. The period is either too excessive while it lasts or continues for a longer time than is normal for that woman. It is generally accompanied by a sense of oppression in the head and lower abdomen, cold feet, chilliness, impaired appetite, and a feeling of lassitude.

Irregular Periods. The periods become irregular and may be extremely heavy or very scanty.

Menopause

Many women going through menopause experience a number of troublesome symptoms involving physiological and emotional changes in varying degrees, but the most prevalent complaint is that of hot flashes. Few women escape this discomfort, although the intensity varies considerably. Generally there is a sudden sensation of heat and flushing particularly of the face. In severe cases this is accompanied by profuse sweating, especially if the woman is very tired or worn out.

Medical authorities explain that the flushing is due to glandular changes which temporarily disturb the balance of the blood. Since glandular upset in the body is likely to cause emotional reactions, it is understandable that many women at this point may overreact to small annoyances, brood over feeling slighted or misunderstood, be given to outbursts of excitability and anger, or become irritable and not speak or answer civilly. Some of the other symptoms of menopause are faintness, cold hands and feet, backaches, insomnia, headaches, and constipation. Another development is poor metabolism resulting in a tendency to gain weight.

NATURAL REMEDIES FOR FEMALE PROBLEMS

The following herbs are used for relieving the symptoms of PMS, menstrual dysfunctions, and menopause.

AGNUS CASTUS

Botanical Name: *Vitex agnus castus*
Common Name: Chaste Tree, Chaste Bush, Nunswort

This lovely tree grows along the shores of the Mediterranean and derives its name from the Greek *Magnos* and the Latin *castus*, both words meaning "chaste." Although there is no mention of this remarkable plant in the old European herbals, it was well known in early Egyptian and Arabian medicine and was credited with valuable healing properties.

Remedial Uses of Agnus Castus

Medical herbalists regard agnus castus as Nature's alternative to chemical drugs for the hormone imbalance of PMS, for menstrual troubles, and for menopause. The plant has gained a well-deserved reputation for alleviating hot flashes, menopausal melancholia, and other problems associated with the change of life. It also reportedly alleviates profuse menstruation, persistent between-periods bleeding, menstrual cramps, absence of periods, recurrent mastitis, and symptoms of PMS.

Scientific Evaluation of Agnus Castus

When a plant's constituents are found to successfully treat various menstrual disorders caused by a deficiency of the luteal hormone, it seems reasonable to assume that the plant may contain the hormone in question. Agnus castus was found so effective in treating PMS, menstrual problems, and menopausal difficulties that research workers in Germany examined the herb by every possible method to determine if its components contain an equivalent of the luteal hormone. When biological and chemical techniques failed to reveal such a hormone, the researchers were convinced that the plant's alkaloids or its other components were producing an effect on the body's glandular system from a higher level.

After further exhaustive studies, the Department of Gynecology at the University of Gottingen concluded that although not a source of the hormone itself, agnus castus has the power to correct and regulate the hormone balance in women through its influence on the pituitary gland.

How Agnus Castus Works

Experts explain that the volatile oil of agnus castus acts on the anterior pituitary gland and shifts the estrogen-progesterone balance toward a "corpus luteum hormone effect."[1] Excess of the follicle-stimulating hormone which is responsible for PMS neurosis is corrected. Also, insufficiency of the luteal-stimulating hormone which causes menorrhagia (profuse menstrual bleeding) is corrected.

The herb also reportedly acts as a precursor (i.e., it combines with certain substances in the body to produce hormones, especially the female group). It does this in a way similar to the way that the provitamin A known as carotene can cause the production of true vitamin A. When the appropriate stimulus is provided, the body can synthesize its own biological molecular compounds and enzymes. In other words, it encourages the body's glandular system to produce its own hormones, and it does this from its own resources.

It has also been discovered that when agnus castus is given for gynecological troubles, unexplained improvements have been observed in cases of shingles and acne vulgaris.

Some Impressive Case Studies

"After taking agnus castus tablets my inter-menstrual bleeding has disappeared and my last period was normal, after eighteen months of misery and inconvenience. Incidentally, not only has my pre-menstrual tension lessened considerably but I also found that my emotions seem to be more balanced.

"I hope many more women will try, and benefit from this marvellous tablet." —Miss A. J.[2]

"After suffering from pre-menstrual tension and dysmenorrhea for a few years, agnus castus tablets worked wonderfully."Mrs. F. D.[3]

"While on a holiday I visited a health food store in an effort to find some relief from menopausal problems, especially hot flashes. The manager recommended agnus castus tablets. They were an instant success. Within a week, I felt better than I had for two years." —Mrs. M. H.[4]

"My friend's daughter had menstrual troubles all her life and would even faint in the middle of giving a lecture at a university. She read about agnus castus and obtained some. The next month, she didn't even know she was starting a period." —Mr. J. A.

"I am 24. After not having a period for five years I took agnus castus tablets. Three months later menstruation took place." —Miss R. S.

"I have been using agnus castus tablets for about a year and have found them remarkably effective in healing the condition of amenorrhea. I believe I should continue taking them until I have established a regular menstrual cycle, and therefore will order a further supply." —H. G.

"The migraine problem is still with me but much improved with agnus castus. Certainly I now have no pre-menstrual tension—a great benefit. Here's hoping I go on improving." —J. R.[5]

"I am very pleased to be able to tell you that agnus castus was an excellent help for my usually painful periods. I didn't experience anything like the pain of previous months." —Mrs. D.

"A dear friend of mine suffered severely from PMS. I suggested she try taking capsules of agnus castus for several days before the start of her monthly period, as that remedy cured me when I had the same distressing problem. She did so, and her PMS suffering is now a thing of the past." —C. T.

BALM

Botanical Name: *Melissa officinalis*
Common Names: Lemon Balm, Sweet Balm, Melissa, Bee Balm

This member of the mint family is a well-known garden plant. When fresh it has a strong lemony aroma and was used in earlier times as a stewing herb to impart a delicate fragrance throughout the home. The botanical name *Melissa* comes from the Greek word for honey. The ancient Greeks placed sprigs of balm in bee hives to attract a swarm, as bees are particularly fond of the herb.

Although balm grows wild in fields and along roadsides, it is the cultivated variety that is used in herbal medicine.

Medicinal Uses

Balm is classified as antispasmodic, calmative, emmenagogue, carminative, and diaphoretic. Its uses in herbal medicine are many, but it is especially valued as a soother of nerves and a reliever of tensions, especially for women troubled by the stress of PMS or by the emotional upset that may accompany menstrual or menopausal problems. Balm is also used to ease menstrual cramps, and as an emmenagogue it is recommended in cases of delayed menstruation.

The tea is prepared by placing 2 teaspoons of the cut herb in a cup of boiling water. The cup is covered with a saucer and allowed to stand for 10 minutes and is then strained.

For suppressed menstruation or menstrual cramps, drink the tea hot, one cup as needed.

For its calming influence in nervous conditions, a cold infusion is prepared with 1-1/2 ounces of balm to 1-1/2 pints of cold water and is left to stand for 12 hours. The infusion is then strained and taken throughout the day, one small wineglass per dose.

If a tincture is used, 1/2 teaspoon is taken in a small glass of water three or four times a day.

SAGE

Botanical Name: *Salvia officinalis*
Common Names: Garden Sage, Meadow Sage, True Sage

The common garden sage is a well-known culinary herb used especially in poultry dressings and sauces for fish. It is a fuzzy perennial plant reaching about 2-1/2 feet in height, bearing blue flowers variegated with purple or white. The flowering time is July to September.

Former Uses

In herbal lore sage was venerated as a sacred herb capable of increasing the life span and was used for so many different ailments that a fourteenth century writer asked, "How can a man die who has sage in his garden?" According to Hippocrates, it was "written that after a pestilence the people of Egypt were told to drink sage tea to make women fertile and thus replenish the population."

To assist digestion, sage was added to sweetmeats following a heavy meal. Cardiac cordials were once made of sage flowers mixed with cinnamon and brandy. The plant was also used for night sweats. To preserve health, country folks used sage as a spring tonic and ate quantities of the leaves in sandwiches with cheese and butter.

Modern Uses of Sage

Sage is classed as aromatic, antihydrotic, antispasmodic, and astringent. One of its best actions is said to be the reduction of excessive perspiration. Generally the reduction begins approximately two hours after taking sage tea or tincture and may last for several days. Scientific experiments were described by Kocher in which he succeeded in almost entirely counteracting the profuse sweating produced by a drug called *pilocarpine* by the administration of sage extracts. This property of sage makes it useful for relieving night sweats and other conditions (e.g., the excessive sweating of menopausal hot flashes).

Sage tea is also recommended for nervousness, trembling, and depression. It is said to be very helpful, too, in conditions of amenorrhea and dysmenorrhea.

The tea is prepared as an infusion—1 teaspoonful of sage is placed in a cup, and boiling water is added. This is allowed to stand for 5 or 10 minutes and is then strained. For troublesome symptoms of menopause, one cup is taken cold at night before retiring. Or two cups of the cold tea may be taken a teaspoonful at a time throughout the day. For amenorrhea or dysmenorrhea, one cup of the tea is taken hot, once or twice a day.

If a tincture is used instead for any of the problems cited, 15 to 40 drops are taken in a little water three or four times a day.

TANG-KUEI

Botanical Name: *Angelica sinensis-polymorpha*
Common Name: Dong Quai

This perennial plant grows from 2 to 3 feet high and is called either tang-kuei or dong quai, depending on the variations of dialects in different parts of China. It has been used by the Chinese since the earliest times and was recorded in *The Herbal* by Shen-Nung.

Remedial Uses

Tang-kuei is employed for treating the symptoms of PMS and menopause and for menstrual aberrations (e.g., dysmenorrhea, scanty periods, stoppage of normal periods, and menstrual irregularity).

Capsules of powdered tang-kuei are available from most health food stores and herb firms. For PMS and menstrual difficulties, two tang-kuei capsules are taken three times daily for 7 to 10 days before the expected menstrual period. The capsules are swallowed with a small glass of water either one-half hour before meals or two hours after.

For menopausal problems, two capsules of tang-kuei are taken twice daily. They may be swallowed with water or broken open and the powder added to broths.

Note. The Chinese use only the best quality of tang-kuei, which has a strong aroma and taste unlike the poorer qualities, which have a faint odor and taste.

Case Studies Highlight Tang-Kuei's Power

"I am 52 years old and I had hot flashes so often I thought I'd go out of my mind. For the past two months I have used Chinese dong quai and the results have been marvelous. Within a few weeks there were no more hot flashes. You cannot imagine what a relief this has been for me." —T. W.

"Chinese tang-kuei is a superb remedy for retarded menstruation. It worked wonders for me when nothing else did." —L. T.

"A teenage girl missed her monthly period for six months. She had been taken to a medical doctor, but her condition did not improve. Her parents were very worried and finally took her to a Chinese herbalist, who prescribed a bottle of dong quai capsules. A few days later the parents went back to the herbalist and happily reported that their daughter's period had started. They saw him again a year later and informed him that the young girl had never had any further trouble with her periods." —L. S.

"The pains of menstrual cramps have vanished since taking herbal capsules of tang-kuei. This has convinced me that no woman ever need suffer monthly cramps when this simple remedy is available." —K. P.

Combined Formula

Tang-kuei is often combined with other herbs for menstrual or menopausal disorders. For example, one formula is called Tang-kuei and Cyperus. It has also been given the name of Nu-shen-san, which means "woman's god," because the remedy is reportedly so effective in relieving menopausal problems. The herbal combination consists of tang-kuei, atractolodes, coptis, cyperus, rhubarb, saussurea, ginseng, areca seed, cinnamon, scute, cnidium, licorice, and clove. This formula is available in capsules.

CRAMP BARK

Botanical Name: *Viburnum opulus*
Common Names: Squaw Bush, Guelder Rose, High Cranberry, Snowball Tree

Cramp bark is a large shrub, growing from 5 to 10 feet high, and belongs to the same family as the elder tree. The snow-white flowers are 3 to 5 inches across, but the inner ones, which provide the nectar for bees, are very small. The fruits, which ripen very quickly, form a drooping cluster of bright red berries, giving the bush a beautiful appearance. Although the berries resemble true cranberries, they are too bitter to be considered palatable.

Medicinal Uses

Cramp bark is classed as antispasmodic and nervine. The active principal of the bark is the bitter glucoside *viburnine*; it also contains resin, tannin, and valeranic acid.

In herbal practice the bark is prepared as a decoction or used in the form of a fluid extract. It has been employed for nervous complaints and debility and used with success in painful spasmodic ailments, especially painful menstrual cramps. Ten to 20 drops of the fluid extract in a little warm water taken three or four times daily has reportedly eased the most painful monthly periods. The same treatment has proved successful in cases of low back pain, especially of uterine origin.

If a decoction is used, it is prepared with 1 teaspoon of the bark to 1 pint of boiling water. This is simmered slowly for 10 minutes and then strained. For severe cramps, the tea is taken hot, one-half to one small teacupful three or four times a day.

LADY'S MANTLE

Botanical Name: *Alchemilla vulgaris*
Common Names: Lion's Foot, Bear's Foot, Nine Hooks

Lady's mantle belongs to the same family as parsley piert. It is an inconspicuous plant about 1 foot high with numerous small flowers, yellow-green in color. The generic name *Alchemilla* is derived from the Arabic word *Alkemelych* (alchemy) in reference to the herb's healing powers.

Remedial Uses

Lady's mantle is classed as astringent, styptic, tonic, and febrifuge. Its healing potential is said to benefit women most. In modern herbal treatment it is employed for excessive menstruation, womb trouble, and menopausal melancholia.

For excessive menstruation, one-half to a teaspoonful extract of lady's mantle is taken in a small glass of water three times a day. Or an infusion may be prepared with 1 ounce of the herb or leaves to 1 pint of boiling water. As soon as the water boils, the container is immediately removed from the burner, allowed to stand for 10 minutes, and then strained. One cupful is taken as needed.

RELEAF™: NATURE'S GIFT TO WOMEN

An herbal product called Releaf™ is manufactured for the Women's Health Institute. It is indicated for the relief of symptoms of PMS such as mood swings (irritability, depression, mental tension), breast tenderness and pain, water retention, abdominal bloating and fatigue. It is also considered effective for relieving menstrual cramps.

The active ingredient in the product is 5 milligrams of vitamin B_6 per capsule combined with a base of the following herbs: wood betony (*Betonica officinalis*), bark of bayberry (*Myrica cerifera*), uva-ursi (*Arctostaphylos uva-ursi*), capsicum (*Capsicum frutescens*), and hawthorn (*Crataegus oxyacantha*).

The formula reportedly contains no aspirin, acetominophen, caffeine, sugar, starch, artificial colors, flavors, or preservatives. It does not cause drowsiness.

How Releaf Is Used

Releaf is available in easy-to-swallow capsules of 365 milligrams each. Three capsules are swallowed with 8 to 10 ounces of water on an empty stomach in the morning, and again with the same amount of water in the evening, making a total of six capsules daily. The capsules are taken every day for six days prior to the onset of menstruation and for two days after menstruation begins. This makes the course of the treatment a total of 48 capsules.

Some Impressive Case Studies

Mrs. D. J. suffered from PMS for 20 years. Her friends described her as having a calm, loving disposition, but for several days before the onset of menstruation it required all her energy to keep a positive frame of mind. She says, "Ask my best friend as she is the one who always kept me sane through it."

Mrs. D. J. had tried every product on the market, including hormone therapy prescribed by a woman gynecologist. Nothing worked. But recently all that changed when she heard about the herbal Releaf formula and decided to try it. She writes: "It happened to be six days before my period. I was just starting to feel edgy. I bought a bottle of Releaf and followed through like the directions recommended. I was astounded. No PMS! None, nada, nothing! A miracle! What Releaf did for my mind and body definitely boosted my spirits. Releaf is not only a product that really works, it is also very easy to take."

Mrs. S. G. writes:"In the past 10 years I have been plagued with PMS—never really knowing what was wrong with me until the last five. I do believe that PMS had a lot to do with my marriage breaking up (hindsight), six years ago. At that point, I was very unhappy but really had no reason to be. I had everything I wanted—a husband who loved me, a bright child who was doing well in school, and a good job. PMS was not really discussed then. I can remember my husband asking me over and over to tell him what he could do to make me happy. I never had an answer."

Mrs. S. G. suffered so severely from PMS that she says she also came close to losing her job because of it. After hearing of several women with the same condition who had used Releaf with excellent results, she decided to try the product. She continues:

"On Sunday, October 30, I started getting depressed and a little edgy. I took three capsules and didn't think about it again. Later that morning a 'friend' called and we had a terrible argument. When I got off the phone I remember walking past my bedroom mirror and I was smiling. It was then I realized that the product works. I normally would have been furious for hours, if not the rest of the day. I can't really tell exactly how soon it worked because it does such a smooth job you forget you even had PMS.

"The following Wednesday I started menstruation and that evening I began having bad cramping. I took four of the herbal capsules and lay down with my feet elevated. Normally, elevating the feet doesn't work for cramping, but in about an hour, maybe a little less, my cramps were gone:

"I know many women who are troubled with the same symptoms of PMS—depression, mood swings, anger, and pain. I want to share with them the knowledge of this remarkable product."

Another young woman reports: "A coworker suggested I try capsules of Releaf for menstrual cramps the next time I got my period. I was sure the herbal capsules wouldn't work, as nothing ever seemed to work for that. I was given three capsules, and I saved them at home until I started my period, on a Friday night. It was the night before my brother-in-law's wedding. I was angry because I knew how I would feel the next day. When I woke up, I was right—I felt like staying home in bed. I remembered the herbal capsules given to me, so I thought I might as well try them. After I took one capsule I showered and got ready for the wedding, and I felt fine the whole day:

"Another time, I was at work and I felt like going home because I had cramps so bad. I felt sick to my stomach because they were so severe. My coworker gave me a few more of her herbal Releaf capsules, and I was just fine.

"I can't believe how well they work. I never found any product that really got rid of menstrual cramps. Releaf really works wonders for me."

One man reported that his wife tried the Releaf formula for PMS and was delighted with the results. He said she only had to take two doses and her symptoms disappeared. Her sister experienced the same beneficial response, and both women agreed that the formula "works like magic."

Mrs. K. tells of a trial run she conducted with the use of Releaf for some of her friends. She writes:

"(1) Carolyn has tremendous depression with PMS. She said she felt great relief after taking three capsules. (2) Peg has depression plus a lot of irritability with PMS, and she said she especially noted that the crabbiness subsided. (3) Margaret is a crab, gets depressed, and retains fluid with PMS. She said she felt 'normal.'

"All the women were aware that the course of treatment would have been a total of 48 capsules, yet all felt relief after one dose of three capsules."

SUMMARY

1. A growing number of medical researchers have presented convincing evidence that PMS is not an imaginary condition but a physically based illness attributed to hormonal imbalances.

2. The symptoms of PMS occur repeatedly for six to eight days or more prior to the onset of menstruation and generally improve after the menses begin.

3. If the symptoms of PMS continue throughout the entire month, the condition is not PMS but something else.

4. Menstruation causes some discomfort for the majority of young women. However, the most common problems are

menstrual cramps, delayed menstruation, cessation of periods, profuse menstrual bleeding, and irregular monthly periods.

5. Women going through menopause experience difficulties in varying degrees, but the most prevalent complaint is hot flashes.

6. Nature has provided a good selection of herbal alternatives to chemical drugs for relieving the symptoms of PMS, menstrual dysfunctions, and menopause.

ENDNOTES

1. Weiss, 1974. *New Herbal Practitioner*, 322, March 1977.
2. *Grace*, Autumn 1982.
3. *Grace*, Spring 1989.
4. *Grace*, Autumn 1987.
5. *Grace*, Spring 1984.

CHAPTER 4

HERBS FOR RHEUMATISM, ARTHRITIS, AND RELATED AILMENTS

Plant remedies along with proper nutritional support have consistently been credited with relieving or eliminating various forms of arthritis and rheumatism. In this chapter we will examine some of these herbal aids.

CHAPARRAL

Botanical Name: *Larrea divaricata*
Common Names: Gobernadora, Creosote Bush, Greasewood

Chaparral is a dark, olive-green shrub which grows in blistering hot, dry, desert regions of the Southwest where few animals or plants can survive. It develops a tap root which reaches 5 or 6 feet in the earth, along with a large network of roots which penetrate 20 feet into the soil and spread out into a wide area. The pulpy bark of the root acts as a reservoir to store water for the plant's use during the drought season. Nature has provided chaparral with varnish-coated tiny leaves to seal in the precious stores of water and also to resist the wind-swept sand storms.

Early Uses

The Indians of the Southwest understood the remarkable healing powers of chaparral long before white people ever arrived in the New World. Due to dietary limitations and the hardships of spending much of their time during the long winter and rainy seasons in damp. smoky dwellings, the Indians suffered severely from arthritis and rheumatism. These painful ailments prompted the natives to search for a variety of remedies, and there is ample evidence that one of the most successful treatments came from chaparral.

The Maricopas heated the fresh twigs over a fire for applications to treat rheumatic pains, and they drank decoctions prepared from the plant to treat conditions of arthritis. Some tribes used the tops of the bush as hot poultices for relieving bodily aches and pains. Others drank teas of the leaves for muscular aches and stiffness and for painful, swollen joints. The herb was also used for treating bruises, tumors, stomach ailments, and pulmonary and throat complaints.

Faith in the healing virtues of chaparral was shared by the Mexicans, who named the herb gobernadora, "the governess" (of the body), because it reputedly cured so many ailments. They also called the plant hediondilla, "the little bad smeller," as the herb has a strong, disagreeable, resinous odor.

Chaparral: A Time-Honored Remedy

In 1848, Dr. J. M. Bigelow, surgeon of the U.S.-Mexican boundary commission, brought the herb to the attention of the medical profession. He reported that a decoction made by boiling the branches and leaves of gobernadora would result in an effective liniment for rheumatism and bruises.

The United States Bulletin, Trees and Shrubs of Mexico[1] states with reference to chaparral that "the plant is much used in domestic medicine, especially for rheumatism, a decoction of the leaves being employed for baths and fomentations. The decoction is said, also, to have remarkable antiseptic properties and is applied to bruises and sores."

The following news item was reprinted in a health publication:[2]

HOPE FOR ARTHRITIS VICTIMS

Chicago—Doctors across the nation are looking at the results researchers are announcing, involving the use of a lowly desert herb in the treatment of stomach ailments, arthritis, and related problems. The plant is the creosote bush, or chaparral, also known as greasewood, and is a member of the oak family.

All tests on chaparral indicate that it is positively non-toxic and has never shown any side effects on patients and if present research is successful it will offer the first anti-cancer drug.

The Indians have used chaparral herb for many internal body malfunctions as well as for rash and acne-type skin eruptions, for hundreds of years.

Constituents in Chaparral

Chaparral has antibiotic and antiseptic properties along with immune stimulating substances. It also contains an important ingredient known as *nordihydroguiaretic* acid (NDGA), a powerful antioxidant and antitumor agent.

Case Studies

Mr. H. K. gives the following impressive accounts of his many years of experience with the use of chaparral:

"The man I work for is like a brother to me, and he grew up at mines his father ran. This was in Mexico, where he learned from the natives many Indian secrets including the healing qualities of this herb (chaparral). On trips with him through the deserts of California and Arizona, to mines he supervised, I was shown the bushes from which to strip the leaves. We would gather a few bushels and bring them back home. I'd brew the tea by the gallons to keep on hand for anyone suffering from arthritis. In the 13 years I've been doing this, I've heard countless people tell how very much the tea has done to reduce swelling and relieve pain, and often to cure."

My Own Case

"After five years in Inglewood, I developed pain in my back and hip areas and eventually could scarcely get up out of a chair alone. Soon I couldn't roll over in bed without breathtaking stabs of pain. I thought I had a diseased kidney or some other organ infected and feared an operation which I could not afford in time or money. Finally I had to have a complete clinical checkup. I was utterly dumbfounded when an orthopedic surgeon looked at all the tests and X-rays and not only told me I had arthritis but that it was too far advanced for any treatment.

"We actually don't know what causes arthritis or how to cure it," he said. "There are all sorts of pills at various prices to experiment with, but frankly, they won't help you. My advice is to make up your mind to live with this as gracefully as you can. Get as much rest as possible and take aspirin to hold down the pain.

"My spine was frozen by calcification, caused by three falls I'd had over many years, down a ship hatch and down mine shafts. I came home and started taking the herb tea that had helped so many others. After a few weeks, I was relatively free from pain. I kept taking it for six months or so and had chiropractic treatments to break the vertebrae loose. I was cured, if that means freedom from all pain, being able to lift anything, to crawl under my truck, jack up and remove wheels, and do other work. I still occasionally take some tea, just to play it safe.

"I take gallons of the tea, free, to a doctor I know as a friend. He puts it in 8 ounce bottles for patients. His own uncle, age 85, had for 15 years been confined to the house, getting around with canes, in severe pain from swollen knees. For those 15 years the doctor tried every medicine that came out, but with no benefit to the sufferer. After taking two bottles of the herb tea, the old man put his canes away; after a few months he was walking all over town to see what he had missed, for he had previously been unable even to ride in an automobile.

"One day at the post office I met Mr. Jones, who lives near me but whom I'd never met before. He had made his first trip to the post office this warm, sunny morning near Christmas, shuffling along slowly. He couldn't even bend over, and his fingers were stiff and enlarged. I drove him home and gave him two bags of gobernadora herbs (which makes 2 to four quarts of tea). In January I took him two more. In March, when I went to his house, I found him outdoors in the flower garden with his wife, weeding. I laughed and kidded him. He stood up and put his arms over his head, stooped down and touched the ground three times. 'I feel like a kid again!' he exclaimed as he showed me his nimble fingers. He stopped taking the tea after two months; it wasn't needed any more.

"You needn't feel hopeless if your arthritis and other similar ills are so bad that the doctors have given up. This herbal cure has been used for thousands of years. It is ancient, but it is still effective."

Instructions for Preparing and Using the Tea

Put 3 ounces of the herb in a pan with a lid, wash in cold water, and drain. Cover with 1 quart plus 1 cup of cold, warm, or hot water. Boil under cover for 5 to 15 minutes as you wish. Let cool enough to put in a glass jar; seal and refrigerate. Just as tea drinkers like to use the same teabag for a second cup of equally good tea, pour another quart of water over the herbs and boil again; then pour off so as to have 2 quarts of tea from the herbs. Fill a small bottle or jar for easy handling after meals.

If you are under a doctor's care, you will ask his or her advice, of course. Most arthritics who use these herbs have either given up doctoring or have been given up as hopeless by doctors and clinics as was I. If you are active enough to eat well, start with 1 teaspoon of the herb tea after one meal a day, your heaviest meal. Increase at your own pace to the same amount after two meals, then to three meals a day. Then increase the amount to two teaspoonsful, and keep raising the dose to 2 ounces after each meal (6 tablespoons). I prefer putting it in canned pineapple-grapefruit juice. Holding your nose as you drink it helps a lot. If you are easily nauseated, start with half a teaspoon until used to it.

Chaparral Tablets

Due to the strong odor and obnoxious taste of chaparral tea, many people prefer to use the herb in tablet form. These are easy to take and are swallowed with a glass of water.

There are several types of chaparral tablets on the market which reportedly give good results, but the best possible qualities are those in which the pure powdered herb leaves are compressed into tablet form without the use of coatings, fillers, binders, excipients, or flavors. The tablet should have a pure herbal aroma. Such tablets are said to preserve the potency and values of natural chaparral as found in the desert.

A Sampling of Additional Case Studies

"After years of agonizing pain of osteoarthritis, I am pain free as a result of taking two 7-1/2 grain chaparral tablets three times daily." —Mrs. S. C.

"There is a man I know who went on a business trip to Mexico City. His wife had painful arthritis which was so bad she had difficulty walking and dressing. Her husband brought home some herbs called gobernadora, which were sold in Mexican shops. He said the herb tea had cured some people in Mexico of rheumatism and arthritis and that his wife is just about cured, too, since taking it." —C. P.

"Last year for months I suffered painful fibrositis in my upper back and shoulder. Weeks of conventional medical treatment were unsuccessful. Toward the end of the year I heard about chaparral and bought a supply of 15-grain tablets, which I took three times a day. There was some relief in a short time, and this encouraged me to continue taking the tablets. Then something happened that I scarcely believed could happen—the pain in my back and shoulder, which almost drove me out of my mind, was gone." —E. T.

"I suffered arthritic joints with much pain and lameness. Cortisone and other medications helped, but I had to stop taking them because of side effects and had eventually even to stop aspirin for the same reason. I tried many other types of therapies, including osteopathic treatments, special diets, and so on, to no avail.

"My husband thought a change of climate might help, so we moved to Arizona. Still there was no improvement in my condition, and I was afraid I'd soon end up in a wheelchair.

"One day, a local resident told me of an Indian herbal remedy known as creosote bush, or chaparral. She said it was a desert plant and that she personally knew of several people who suffered from arthritis who had been helped, and some cured, with its use.

"I tried the tea but couldn't stand the terrible taste, so I used the tablets, one 15-grain tablet at each meal and one at bedtime.

"Within two weeks, the pain had mercifully subsided. It was like a miracle. I have been taking the tablets daily for three months and am 90% free of arthritis. There is no more lameness or pain, and except for a slightly stiff neck, I feel just wonderful." —J. P.

GOUTWORT

Botanical Name: *Aegopodium podagraria*
Common Names: Gout Herb, Bishopwort, Bishopsweed, Goutweed

Goutwort is native to almost all European countries and to Russian Asia. It is a common weed seen in the outskirts of villages and towns and is considered a pest in the garden.

The herb was given the common names of bishopswort and bishopsweed because it was often seen growing near old monastery ruins. It is claimed that the plant was introduced by the monks of the Middle Ages, who cultivated it for use as a healing agent.

As the popular name of goutwort implies, the herb was used for painful gouty conditions. The same implication can also be seen in the botanical name *podagraria*, which was taken from the Latin *podagra*, meaning "gout."

A Brief Definition of Gout

Gout is defined as a disorder of the purine metabolism of the body. Instead of the body's waste products, known as uric acid crystals, being filtered out of the blood, they are deposited in and around the joints and cause the surrounding cartilage and tendons to become inflamed. An attack can occur suddenly, accompanied by severe pain.

Remedial Uses of Goutwort

Goutwort is classed as diuretic and sedative. Medical herbalists still regard the herb as an effective remedy for treating gout, neuritis, and aches and pains in the joints. It is also used for sciatica, a condition in which the sciatic nerve and its branches are affected, with the pain extending from the area of the buttocks to the back of the thigh and leg. (When one or more nerve trunks in other parts of the body become inflamed, the condition is known as neuritis.)

For any of these disorders, a tea is prepared by pouring 1 pint of boiling water into an enamel pot containing 1 ounce of goutwort leaves. The pot is covered with a lid and the tea is allowed to stand for five minutes and is then strained.

In chronic cases, one teacupful is taken four or five times a day; in acute cases it is taken every two hours until relieved. If the fluid extract is used instead, one-half to a teaspoonful is taken in a small glass of water three times a day.

Accessory Treatments for Gout, Sciatica, and Neuritis

Gout. During an acute attack of gout, rest is usually indicated. If the joint of the toe or knee is affected, it is advisable to have the foot or leg slightly elevated and resting on cotton batting to help ease the pain.

Herbalists advise sufferers of gout to drink plenty of water and to keep the bowels open. The diet should be light, and purine foods should be avoided. These include such foods as chocolate, smoked salmon, shellfish, and some meats (e.g., veal, liver, lamb, sweetbreads, heart, and all forms of pork). Alcoholic beverages, especially beer and red wines, are also on the forbidden list.

Some examples of foods fairly free of purines are vegetables, milk, cereals, cheese, and white fish such as halibut or cod. Buttermilk is especially recommended. As one medical herbalist explains:

> Inasmuch as gouty difficulties arise from sluggish excretion, buttermilk is a blessing to all gouty subjects. The lactic acid, the 'sour' of the buttermilk, attacks and dissolves

all sorts of deposits in the blood vessels. If anyone has a creaky joint or a swollen and aching one, he should drink all the buttermilk he can relish whenever and wherever he can. A quart a day should be the minimum according to taste.

Sciatica. Conditions of painful sciatica reportedly respond very well to the use of goutwort poultices. To prepare the poultice, the leaves and roots of goutwort are boiled together slowly for five minutes and then spread evenly on a piece of cloth. The cloth is folded over once and applied hot to the large muscle of the buttock. The poultice is covered with a piece of wax paper and a dry towel to retain the heat. As soon as the poultice begins to cool, it is steeped again in the hot water and reapplied. The method is continued until relief is obtained.

Neuritis. Hot poultices of goutwort also bring relief in conditions of neuritis. If the pain is in the shoulder, arm, or fingers, the poultice is applied to the top of the spine in line with the collar bone. The poultice has a soothing effect on the inflamed nerve where it branches out from the spine.

Herbalists encourage those suffering from neuritis or sciatica to include liberal amounts of unpolished brown rice in their diets. This recommendation is well founded, as unpolished brown rice contains minerals and vitamins among which are the major B vitamins known as the antineuritis vitamins. A deficiency of these essential elements tends to bring on the condition of neuritis or sciatica.

YUCCA

Botanical Name: *Yucca glauca*
Common Names: The Lord's Candle, Soapweed

Yucca is a hardy plant which thrives in hot, dry climates and in sandy soil. Masses of aromatic, bell-shaped white flowers burst into bloom from the thick stalk, which grows from the center of the plant and rises to a height of about 10 feet. Because of this beautiful flowering, the plant was often called the Lord's Candle.

Yucca has long been used for healing and practical purposes by the American and Mexican Indians.

Constituents in Yucca

Scientists have discovered that yucca roots contain a high concentration of saponins, natural substances which are similar to steroids such as cortisone. Some researchers have demonstrated that yucca saponin extracts in tablet form relieve the swelling and pain for many arthritics and also produce a beneficial effect on bursitis and rheumatism. It also has been indicated that the extract improves digestion and reduces the tendency to accumulate toxic wastes in the colon.

Reported Uses

The use of yucca tablets has relieved many cases of bursitis, a condition in which the bursa (a small, semifluid sac which is formed around a joint and acts as a cushioning device) becomes irritated or inflamed. For example, a 63-year-old woman could scarcely raise her left arm because of bursitis of the shoulder joint accompanied by inflammation of the tendons. At the end of 21 days of taking two yucca tablets three times daily, she was symptom free and has had no further attacks in two years. A 50-year-old man had bursitis of the shoulder joint for two-and-a-half months. Pain was relieved in one week after taking two yucca tablets twice a day, and within 14 days he had normal pain-free movement of the joint. In another case a 47-year-old woman developed bursitis of the knee. She took three yucca tablets daily for two weeks, then one tablet a day thereafter. She reports that the pain was noticeably reduced within four days and completely eliminated in less than three weeks. In still another case, a 29-year-old man complained of bursitis of the shoulder joint associated with neuralgic pain that radiated down to his hand and fingers. He took two yucca tablets daily for about five days. He then stopped taking the tablets, but the pain returned within 24 hours. The pain disappeared again within several hours after he resumed taking the tablets.

Symptoms did not return after three weeks' use of the tablets.

Accessory Treatment Provides Relief

Heat applied to the area of busitis will usually intensify the pain, but cold compresses or an ice bag generally bring relief until the prescribed herbal treatment can take effect.

TWIN LEAF

Botanical Name: *Jeffersonia diphylla*
Common Names: Rheumatism Root, Ground Squirrel Pea, Yellow Root

This small perennial plant is found in various parts of the United States and grows chiefly in limestone soils, which may account for its age-old reputation as an effective remedy for neuralgia (some cases of this disorder are believed to result from a lack of lime in the system).

Twin Leaf for Trigeminal Neuralgia (Tic Douloureux)

Trigeminal neuralgia is an affection of the fifth cranial trigeminal nerve, which has three branches distributed chiefly to the face, forehead, and jaw. It is characterized by severe pain on one side of the face and tends to occur in paroxysms followed by continuous pain. It is more common in damp, cold climates and is often preceeded by general ill health.

Herbalists advise patients with this condition to avoid drafts to the face and to improve their health by means of diet and herbal tonics. Vitamin B complex has also been found to be beneficial and can be taken in tablet form along with a specific remedy such as twin leaf.

How Twin Leaf Is Used

Twin leaf is prepared in the form of a decoction: One ounce of the root is placed in a saucepan and 1 pint of boiling hot water is added. The brew is allowed to steep (stand) for half an hour and is then simmered slowly for 10 minutes. One cup of the strained decoction is taken, followed later with small, frequent doses.

If the tincture is preferred, the dose is one-half to a teaspoonful in a small glass of water three or four times a day.

Accessory Treatment Reduces Pain

In conditions of facial neuralgia, a hot moist herbal pack is prepared by placing the leaves of twin leaf in a cloth bag and soaking the bag in hot water. When it has been sufficiently wrung out, the pack is applied as hot as can be comfortably borne to the painful area and is then covered with suitable material to retain the heat. In severe cases of facial neuralgia it may take half an hour before the pain becomes noticeably less.

The herbal pack may also be applied to help relieve the pains of rheumatism.

Case Studies

With regard to the use of twin leaf for facial neuralgia, a judge wrote:

"For what it has done for my wife and daughter I would not take thousands of dollars. At times the pain was so bad that it threw them into convulsions. The preparations of the best physicians were used in vain. They found no relief until they tried twin leaf, which acted almost like a charm in curing them.

"I recommended it to a friend who had been suffering for three days and nights with little sleep or rest. One dose of twin leaf gave her immediate relief, followed by 10 hours' sleep."

ELDERBERRY

Botanical Name: *Sambucus canadensis*
Common Names: Pipe Tree, Popgun Tree, Common Elder

The American elder is a shrub bearing small, white flowers and purple-black or red berries. It is found growing in all parts of the country in low, damp ground and thickets.

The word elder comes from the Anglo-Saxon *aeld*, meaning "fire." The name comes from the old practice of removing the pith from the young branches and using them as blowing tubes to kindle fire. Because the tubes were also made into shrill musical pipes,the elder is still frequently called the pipe tree. The shoots with the pith removed were used by youngsters for making popguns.

Traditional Healer

The elder has enjoyed a long reputation for its medicinal virtues. The gypsies referred to it as the "healingest tree on earth." Hippocrates listed it among the prominent plants of his materia medica, and it was also mentioned by Pliny and other ancient writers.

In 1644 a book was written titled *The Anatomy of the Elder*, a treatise of some 230 pages, which deals with the medicinal value of the tree. It sets forth 70 classes of diseases, including rheumatism, and describes the many forms in which the elder is used.

The elder was also well known to the American Indians. The cooked berries were eaten and prepared as a drink for rheumatism, neuralgia, sciatica, and back pain. Some tribes used sweat baths prepared with infusions of elderberry leaves and flowers and at the same time drank hot elderberry tea. They claimed this treatment induced profuse sweating which brought compete relief from the pains of rheumatism.

Health Properties in Elder

Elderberries provide vitamins A, B, and C. *Elderin,* a glucoside which is identical to rutin, is found in the flowers. In addition, they contain a fragrant volatile oil and malates of potash and lime. Other constituents of the plant are pectin, starch, gum fat, resin, grape sugar, and various alkaline and earthy salts. Elderberries contain viburnic acid and a substance which induces perspiration.

As a domestic remedy for the relief of rheumatism, 1 pint of boiling water is poured over 1 ounce of elderberry flowers. The container is then covered and the tea is allowed to stand for five minutes. One cup of the strained tea is taken three or four times daily. This simple tea is very popular in Europe, where the sale of dried elder flowers has increased by 50% during the past several years.

Elderberry for Neuralgia and Sciatica

Back in the old days, cheap port wine was often combined with elderberry juice to resemble expensive dark red port. In 1889, an American sailor informed a physician that drinking port wine was a sure cure for trigeminal neuralgia and sciatica. An investigation resulted in the discovery that the wine was combined with elderberry juice. A series of tests showed that while port wine has practically no pain-relieving properties, the addition of elderberry juice often banishes the pain of sciatica and neuralgia.

Later Studies

Two Prague doctors, Epstein and Jokel, reported on the beneficial aspects of elderberry juice on cases of trigeminal neuralgia. Dr. Epstein had prescribed rubbing the affected area with elderberry wine and was amazed at how quickly the pain subsided. He then began to experiment with pure elderberry juice without any alcohol. Forty-eight patients suffering from painful neuralgia were instructed to drink 20 grams of the juice daily. Dr. Epstein says the results were astonishing. In acute cases the condition often cleared up after only one dose. In chronic cases several days were required before the ailment yeilded to the elderberry treatment. Later, he found that some alcohol (20%) added to the juice was more effective and shortened the period of time required for a complete healing. So convinced was he of the value of his unique treatment that if beneficial results did not occur, he considered the disorder to be other than trigeminal neuralgia. Dr. Jokel's findings confirmed those of Dr. Epstein.

Dr. Vetlesen, a Norwegian, combined 10 grams of port wine with 30 grams of elderberry juice and prescribed this as a daily dose to patients suffering from sciatica. In acute cases the ailment yielded in from 1 to 11 days. In relapsing cases, 23 days' treatment was necessary to establish a complete healing with lasting results. Other European doctors have confirmed these experiences.

Another Case Study

Mrs. M. L. relates her experiences with elderberry wine:

"When I was in my late forties, I started getting acute attacks of facial neuralgia. I would walk the floor all day and half the night with terrible stabbing pains shooting into my right temple and cheek. Then one time when I was suffering from one of these horrible attacks, my husband brought home a bottle of elderberry wine and told me he had heard it was a good remedy for neuralgia.

"Following his advice on how it was to be used, I heated a little of the elderberry wine in a pan and soaked a large piece of cotton in it. Then I bound the cotton on the side of my face and temple and rested in bed. I also drank about a third of a cupful of hot elderberry wine.

"It brought such blessed relief that I soon fell asleep. When I awoke hours later, the pain was gone. For the rest of that day, I remained quietly in bed and drank about one-third of a teacup of the wine three different times to make sure the pain would not return.

"I didn't get another attack until several months later, and I noticed right away that it was not nearly as severe as the attacks once were. I used the elderberry wine remedy again, the same way as before, and got the same wonderful results.

"The elderberry treatment gradually cured me, as I have had no further attacks for the past five years."

AGNUS CASTUS

Botanical Name: *Vitex agnus castus*
Common Names: Chaste Tree, Chaste Bush, Nunswort

Dr. Bartram suggests the use of agnus castus as a possible preventive measure against the development of osteoporosis. He writes:[3]

Osteoporosis affects women more than men. It is a disorder where the bone fabric is lost and is a common cause of women losing height after menopause. A vague backache may be felt as vertebrae become thinner and surrounding nerves are squeezed. It is believed to be a hormonal problem though diet plays an important part. Good wholesome food is essential.

Women at risk of this bone disease are advised to take agnus castus as a continuous hormone replacement aid from the onset of menopause. Doing so may offer some protection to the neck of the femur (the thigh bone, originating in the hip and extending down to the knee).

Women at high risk from osteoporosis are usually those with high intakes of phosphates, protein and particularly caffeine (coffee), of sedentary lifestyle, and who indulge in the smoking habit.

Dr. Bartam adds that agnus castus may be combined with a calcium supplement (1-gram tablet) three times daily.

CHERRY

Botanical Name: *Prunus serotina* and other species
Common Names: Wild Black Cherry, Sweet Cherry, Sour Cherry

The cherry tree is cultivated in most parts of the world but thrives best in temperate climates. In herbal medicine, all parts of the cherry tree—the fruit, leaves, bark, and root—are used for treating many different ailments.

Properties in Cherries

Cherries are excellent sources of vitamins A, B, and C along with an abundance of minerals. They also contain bioflavenoids and pectin. Because of its ability to gel and hold water together, pectin is a powerful blood cleanser. It rids the body of harmful toxins which can leave dangerous deposits and cause diseases such as arthritis and related disorders.

Cherries for Gout

Because of intense suffering from painful gout in his big toe, Ludwig Blau, Ph.D., was confined to a wheelchair. One day when he was at home alone he became hungry, but except for a bowl of cherries almost all the food on hand was too rich in purines for his restricted diet. Having no other recourse, he began eating the cherries.

The next morning he was amazed to find that the pain in his toe was almost gone. He began to wonder if by any chance the cherries he had eaten the day before had anything to do with it. So he decided to test the idea by eating six cherries every day. Before long he was free of pain and back on his feet.

He reports that sometime later when he was out of town, he forgot about the cherries, and in a few days the gout returned. Dr. Blau immediately resumed eating the cherries and experienced the same beneficial results as before. He continued eating from six to eight cherries every day and has remained free of gout.

Dr. Blau reported his first experience with cherries to his physician, who began doing some checking on his own. Before long, there were 12 case histories of gout sufferers who had been relieved by eating cherries or drinking cherry juice. Dr. Blau reported these findings in an article titled "Cherry and Diet Control for Gout and Arthritis."[4] He wrote that the blood uric acid level in the 12 cases of gout had lowered to its usual average, and "no attacks of gouty arthritis have occurred on a *non-restricted* diet in all twelve cases as a result of eating about one-half pound of fresh or canned cherries per day."

Relief was obtained by eating either fresh Black Bing varieties or canned cherries—sour, black or Royal Anne. In one case only the juice was taken and the beneficial results proved to be about equal.

Dr. Blau published the information on the use of cherries for gout so that "it might offer a merciful means of relief to hundreds of thousands of American victims who suffer the agonizingly painful torture that drives many to thoughts of suicide."

Later Evidence

Eight years after Dr. Blau's report was published, an article in the *Food Field Reporter* [5] cited new evidence that gouty arthritis, gout, and similar ailments may be relieved by drinking canned cherry juice. It was reported that the cherry juice was taken by a number of residents of Sturgeon Bay, Wisconsin, who participated in the study. According to the article, "outstanding results were reported."

A Few Tips about Using Cherries

Should you wish to use canned cherries, keep in mind that most brands sold in supermarkets are loaded with sugar and also probably artificial coloring and other chemicals. For maximum benefit, nutritionists recommend organically grown cherries that are bottled or canned without the addition of sugar and chemicals, available from manufacturers of health food store products.

Additional Case Studies

One woman reported that her husband obtained complete relief from gout in his toe and that the pain in his back and shoulders had eased within two days of eating sweet cherries.

Another gout sufferer drank cherry juice daily for one week and reported that the pain in his knee, which had tormented him almost beyond endurance, was gone. He went on to say, "My brother, who suffered from arthritis in his fingers, was so impressed with the results I achieved that he decided to try the cherry juice remedy. After using it for two weeks, he noticed that the pain and swelling in his fingers had lessened. Encouraged by the improvement, he continued drinking cherry juice every day and two months later found he was able to bend his fingers into a fist, something he had not been able to do for some time."

Mr. T. R. suffered periodic attacks of gout for three years. He said the only thing that gave him any relief was "to have the doctor remove fluid from my knee and give me a shot of medicine." One morning he read a news item about the use of cherries for gout, and since there were some sour cherries in the freezer, he began eating a dessert dish of them at lunch and dinner. The swelling in his knee went down, and the stiffness was gone in three days. He continued eating two dishes of the cherries daily and has had no further attacks of gout in over a year.

Mrs. J. L., troubled with gouty arthritis, said she bought some sour cherries to bake a pie but picked at them until she had eaten about one-half pound. She claims that within a few hours the pain in her shoulder and arm had lessened. During the entire fruit season she continued eating the cherries and says she was relieved of her arthritis pain the entire time. However, she found that if she stopped eating the cherries the pain returned. She froze the cherries and resumed eating them and reports that she has been completely free of the arthritis condition for the past 10 years.

Note. If you want to try the variety called "sour cherries," do not be mislead by the name. When the fruit is ripe you'll find it very sweet and flavorful.

SUMMARY

1. The desert herb chaparral, also known as gobernadora and creosote bush, has been used for ages as an effective remedy for some forms of arthritis.

2. Tests on chaparral have shown that it is nontoxic and has no side effects.

3. Those who wish to use chaparral in tea form are advised to start with small amounts, as little as one-half teaspoonful, and gradually work up to the larger doses of 2 ounces after each meal.

4. Mixing chaparral tea with canned fruit juice helps to mask the herb's obnoxious taste, or the herb can be taken in tablet form.

5. In conditions of sciatica, hot herbal poultices are applied to the area of the buttocks and hips; in facial neuralgia they are placed directly on the painful side of the face; in neuritis of the arm they are applied to the top of the spine along the line of the collar bone. These applications are used in conjunction with drinking specific herbal teas.

6. Nutritionists advise sufferers of neuritis and sciatica to include plenty of unpolished brown rice in their diets.

7. Heat applied to bursitis will usually intensify the pain, but cold compresses or an ice bag generally bring relief until the herbal treatment can take effect.

8. Cherries and cherry juice have proved effective in coping with many cases of gout even when a restricted diet is not followed.

ENDNOTES

1. Vol. 23.
2. *Grace,* Autumn 1972.
3. *Grace,* Summer 1988.
4. *Texas Reports on Biology and Medicine,* Vol. 8, No. 3, Fall 1950. November 10, 1958.

CHAPTER 5

HERBS FOR COPING WITH GENITOURINARY PROBLEMS

In his article titled "Kidney Stones Removed by Herbal Medicine—Valuable Treatment by Parsley Piert"[1], Dr. Evans (Naturopathic Doctor, Fellow of the National Institute Medical Herbalists of England) writes:

> I do not know whether there is a law governing coincidence but it was certainly a very propitious moment when my telephone rang and the caller, who had only recently been introduced to natural medicine, began to eulogize the virtues of parsley piert. It was precisely at that moment I was in the process of preparing an article on this particular herb for a medical journal.
>
> My informant described how a stone had become lodged in his right kidney and in spite of treatment by his doctor there was no sign of it moving. The pain was considerable and he was at last advised to have surgical intervention. While examining the possibility of such action a friend suggested that he should try the herbal remedy parsley piert before undergoing hospital treatment. With nothing to lose, the man purchased a quantity of the dried herb which he infused and drank in copious quantities several times a day. Within a fortnight (two weeks) the pain had vanished. His doctor then ordered a second X-ray, the result of which showed nothing visible; the obstruction had disappeared completely. This is only one of the many accounts illustrating the invaluable use of parsley piert for kidney stones.

Let us consider this unique herb and some of the many others that are used in botanic medicine for treating genitourinary problems.

73

PARSLEY PIERT

Botanical Name: *Alchemilla arvensis*
Common Names: Parsley Breakstone, Parsley Piercestone

Parsley piert grows abundantly in fields, waste places, gravel pits, and on the tops of walls. It is a very small plant seldom reaching more than 4 inches high. The tiny greenish flowers are bunched together in tufts and are almost completely hidden by the broad green leaves. Because of its action on stones and gravel in the kidneys and bladder, it was given the common names of parsley breakstone and parsley piercestone.

Note. Parsley piert is not related to the common garden parsley, although its remedial action is somewhat similar.

Medicinal Uses

Parsley piert is classed as diuretic and demulcent. It is chiefly used by herbalists for treating gravel, stones, and urinary ailments.

If the fluid extract of the herb is used, 1 teaspoon is taken in a small glass of water twice a day. Or an infusion may be prepared by placing 1 ounce of the herb in an enamel saucepan with 1 pint of cold water. This is brought to a boil, simmered for one minute, and then set aside until cold. It is then strained, and one teacupful is taken three or four times daily.

Combined Formulas

Parsley piert is sometimes used in combination with other plant diuretics such as buchu, pellitory of the wall, and wild carrot. To soothe and assist the passage of irritating substances, it is often administered with other demulcents (e.g., mullein flowers, sweet flag root, marshmallow root, comfrey root, or slippery elm).

For patients suffering from stones or gravel in the bladder, Dr. Evans recommends the following herbal combination, which he says is very effective:[2]

1 oz. parsley piert

1 oz. pellitory of the wall

1 oz. gravel root

2 oz. marshmallow root

Mix: Bring to a boil in 2-1/2 pints of water. Simmer down to 2 pints. Cool. Strain. Take one wineglassful three times a day. The herbs over this formula will facilitate the dissolution of the stones.

Case Studies Affirm Parsley Piert's Effectiveness

"I suffered severe cutting pains in the lower part of my abdomen in the region of the bladder. At times there was a little blood in the urine. X-rays showed there were several small stones in the bladder, and my doctor told me that the pain from which I suffered was caused by the sharp edges of the stones which lacerated the urinary tract. Surgery was advised, but I was very fearful of going under the knife.

"Fortunately I heard of an herbal formula consisting of parsley piert, marshmallow root, gravel root, and pellitory which was recommended for dissolving bladder stones. After using this tea on a daily basis for some time, X-rays showed there was no longer any trace of the bladder stones." —Mr. D. C.

"Several years ago I suffered a severe attack of cystitis. During the long, painful months that followed, I tried everything medicine had to offer, with only temporary relief. To make matters worse, I was afraid my marriage would break up, as sexual intercourse became almost impossible and my husband was growing more and more irritable with each passing day. In desperation I turned to herbs, and it is to them that I owe my return to health and marital happiness.

"To others who suffer from distressful cystitis I say 'Don't give up hope. Keep trying until you find the remedy that works for you.' In my own case I used the following combination gleaned from a health magazine.

"Mix together 1 ounce of parsley piert and buchu, and 1/2 ounce of wild carrot seeds. Put two heaping teaspoons in a teacup and add boiling water. Let stand until cold. Strain. Take one teacup between meals three times daily. Avoid coffee, alcohol, and peppermint as these interfere with the beneficial effects of the remedy." —Mrs. E. H.

"I am so glad I followed a recommendation to try parsley piert for my wife's dropsy. She has passed a lot of water since." —Mr. J. T.

"Over the years I've had surgery two different times for the removal of kidney stones and was again facing another operation for the same condition. In hopes of avoiding the surgery, I consulted an herbalist, who advised that I drink a tea of parsley piert four times a day. I followed his suggestion, and after a few months or so X-rays gave me a clean bill of health. The herbalist also advised that I take 200 milligrams of vitamin B_6 daily to prevent any further formation of the stones. I have been doing this and have not experienced any more kidney stone attacks in the past eight years." —Mrs. C. C.

Relative to the foregoing case study, a recent study of 100 kidney stone patients was undertaken in India. The patients were treated with vitamin B_6 and it was found that the stones stopped forming in all of them.

Dr. Nortman, a kidney specialist and associate clinical professor of medicine at UCLA, explained that vitamin B_6 interferes with the body's production of oxalic acid, which is involved in forming kidney stones. He said he treats his patients with 200 to 300 milligrams of vitamin B_6 a day to help prevent stone formation.

Dr. David Heber, professor of medicine and chief of the division of clinical nutrition of UCLA, said that you can safely take up to 300 milligrams of vitamin B_6 daily. He pointed out that larger doses may cause side effects, but not at this level.

PIPSISSEWA

Botanical Name: *Chimaphila umbellata*
Common Names: Prince's Pine, False Wintergreen, Ground Holly

Pipsissewa is indigenous to the north temperate regions of both hemispheres. It is a small evergreen perennial with a creeping yellow rhizome which has several erect stems 4 to 8 inches high. The flowers are light purple with cream-colored petals, purplish at the base.

Early Uses

It is apparent from its quaint Algonquin name meaning "breaks into small pieces" (i.e., bladder stones), that pipsissewa was a time-honored remedy of the American Indians. The Catawbas called the plant "fire flower" and used it to treat backache. Other tribes employed it as a tea for urinary disorders, rheumatism, and female problems.

Later the settlers began to use the herb, and it retained its popularity for years before being adopted by the early medical profession. In general, doctors employed decoctions of the herb for intermittent fevers, urinary complaints, and rheumatism.

Modern Remedial Uses

Pipsissewa is classed as alterative, astringent, diuretic, and diaphoretic. It is used by medical herbalists for catarrh of the bladder, urethritis, scalding urine, urinary infections, and kidney problems. It is also considered a good remedy for ascites; however, in conditions of dropsy it is combined with other herbs.

Prolonged use of the leaf tea has been recommended for dissolving bladder stones.

The tea is prepared by placing 1 teaspoon of pipsissewa in a cup and adding boiling water. This is allowed to stand until cold and is then strained. One or two cups of the cold tea are taken daily, a large mouthful at a time.

A Combined Formula

Dr. Swinburne Clymer[3] states that in diseases of the kidneys and in dropsy, "pipsissewa exerts a powerful influence toward a cure." He writes:

> For dropsy combine with populus (poplar bark), mix together:
>
> Tinct. Pipsissewa 1 oz.
>
> Tinct. Populus 1/2 oz.
>
> Dose 15 to 60 drops in plenty of water. The same combination may be given successfully in conditions where the urine is scanty and contains offensive and nonoffensive pus, or pus and blood mixed, or when the urine is scalding or burning; in chronic urethral and prostatic irritation; chronic relaxation of the bladder; and chronic prostatitis with catarrh of the bladder.

Scientific Research on Pipsissewa

Scientific research has shown that pipsissewa possesses antibacterial power. The alcoholic and water extracts have been found to contain in vitro antibiotic activity. Two hundred and nine Nova Scotian plants were tested for antibacterial power against *E. coli* and *Staph. aureus* by Bishop and MacDonald.[4] Pipsissewa was reported to be one of the 10 most active plants.

BUCHU

Botanical Name: *Barosma betulina*
Common Names: Bucku, Bookoo

This small plant is indigenous to South Africa, found chiefly in the vicinity of Cape Town. The natives use the leaves of several species all under the common name of buchu, but the principal variety grown and considered the most valuable is *Barsoma betulina*. The leaves are collected while the plant is flowering and bearing fruit and are then dried and exported.

Buchu was introduced into official medicine in Great Britain in 1821 as a remedy for urethritis and cystitis.

Medicinal Action and Uses

Buchu is classed as a mild antiseptic and antibacterial. It is considered beneficial in the treatment of cystitis, gravel, urethritis, prostatitis, catarrh, and irritation of the bladder.

Buchu may be used either as teas, tablets, powders, fluid extracts, or tinctures. When preparing the tea, it should never be allowed to boil *continuously,* as this would destroy the plant's essential oil responsible for its antiseptic and antibacterial action. One heaping teaspoon of the leaves is placed in a cup, which is then filled with boiling water and covered with a saucer. The tea is allowed to stand until cold and is then strained. One-half to one cup is taken cold, morning and mid-day.

If either the fluid extract or the tincture is used, generally one-half to one teaspoon is taken in a small glass of water twice daily. (Dr. Clymer suggests 10 to 40 drops of the tincture.)

Combined Buchu Formulas

Bed-Wetting A European herbalist recommends the following formula for conditions of bed-wetting in children:

> Fluid extract of buchu 1/2 ounce; fluid extract of marshmallow root 1/2 ounce; fluid extract of agrimony 1 ounce; fluid extract of licorice root 1 drachm (approx. 1 teaspoon). Mix the extracts together and add water to six ounces. Dose: One desertspoonful in water three times daily. Regulate the dose according to age.

Kidney and Bladder Weakness One-half ounce each of buchu, juniper berries, couch grass, and uva-ursi are mixed together and simmered very gently for 15 minutes in 2 pints of water and then strained. One teacupful is taken before meals three times daily.

Case Studies One woman stated that she purchased some buchu tablets for cystitis and found, "they helped immediately." Another woman reported that her friend, the elderly wife of a medical doctor, suffered from chronic cystitis, which modern medicine did not cure. She said, "My friend decided to try buchu extract after reading an article about this unusual herb. In a few weeks, to the amazement of her husband, she was cured."

Mrs. C. writes: "Earlier this year I came down with a bad case of urethritis. After months of disappointing medical treatment, buchu brought wonderful results. I feel like a new person. I thought others should know about this herb remedy."

Another lady reports: "My doctor's prescription for an attack of cystitis (an unusual complaint for me) resulted in very unpleasant effects—a thudding head and a thumping heart, during the night. So I stopped taking them and decided to take buchu compound tablets. I was cured in a week. I am so pleased I have recommended them to a friend."[5]

ERYNGO

Botanical Name: *Eryngium maritinum*
Common Name: Sea Holly

This plant abounds on the sandy seashores in parts of Europe and various other coastal sections of the world. The leaves have a sea-green glossy hue and are veined in white, while the thistle-like flowers which grow at the top of the stem are fringed with blue. The young flowering shoots are said to be palatable and nutritious when boiled and eaten like asparagus. Roasted or boiled, the roots taste like chestnuts and are also considered nutritious.

The roots of eryngo are supposed to contain aphrodisiac properties and are still regarded in some lands as excellent restoratives. In the sixteenth and seventeenth centuries they were candied and sold as "kissing comforts," a reference to their alleged aphrodisiac virtues.

Modern Remedial Uses

Eryngo is classed as diuretic, diaphoretic, expectorant, stimulant, and aromatic. It is mostly used a a remedy for bladder diseases, uterine irritation, dropsy, and painful micturition with frequent ineffective attempts to empty the bladder.

A decoction is prepared with 1 ounce of the root to 1-1/2 pints of boiling water. This is simmered slowly down to 1 pint and then strained. One wineglassful is taken three times daily before meals.

Two Interesting Cases

Dr. Charles Abbott, M.I. Bth, states that for many years he has employed eryngo in various forms with the greatest success in treating his patients. For example, he writes:[6]

> I was called to one of the worst cases of Bright's Disease and dropsy I had ever seen or heard of. The woman was like a huge balloon, The cure had the miraculous touch that only eryngo can give. (The patient was given the following formula.) Mix together:

Fluid extract eryngo 1 oz.

    "   "   holy thistle 1/2 oz.

    "   "   dandelion root 1/2 oz.

    "   "   juniper berries 1/2 oz.

    "   "   yarrow 1/2 oz.

One-half teaspoonful three times a day.

Another case which Dr. Abbott reports involved a 7-year-old boy who had been diagnosed at medical school as suffering from hydrocele (a condition in which fluid collects in the sac surrounding the testicles). The mother was informed that her young son should have surgery, but she decided to contact Dr. Abbott first to see if herbal remedies might help. She was instructed to mix together 1 ounce fluid extract of eryngo and 4 teaspoons fluid extract of comfrey root and to give her son 5 drops of the mixture in a little water three times a day. Dr. Abbott reports:

> At the next School Examination there was much discussion between the M.O. (medical officer) and the nurse and the mother was informed there was nothing to worry about—there wasn't as the hydrocele had disappeared, never to return.

SAW PALMETTO

Botanical Name: *Saba serrulata*
Common Names: Sabal, Palmetto

This plant grows abundantly in the sandy soils of the southwestern coast of the U.S. It is a decumbent-stemmed palm, forming palmetto scrubs which extend for hundreds of miles along the coastline from Georgia to Florida. The berries are about the size of an olive, deep purple in color, and contain a large quantity of juice.

Remedial Uses

Saw palmetto is classed as nutritive, tonic, and diuretic. It is especially prized for treating inflammation of the urinary passage and for its reputed ability to provide nutrients to the testicles and mammae in functional atrophy of these organs.

A tincture of saw palmetto berries combined equally with tincture of echinacea is considered a valuable remedy for enlarged prostate. This was the combination used by Dr. Eric Powell, a naturopathic doctor in England, for treating an elderly man suffering from the disorder. He says that the herbal mixture normalized the patient's prostate gland in three months and adds, "I was particularly pleased with the results in this case owing to his age, for he was over seventy." The mixture was taken in five-drop doses in a little water three times daily before meals.

MEXICAN DAMIANA

Botanical Name: *Turnera aphrodisiaca*
Common Name: Damiana

This is a small shrub with light green, wedge-shaped leaves and aromatic yellow flowers. It is native to northern Mexico, lower California, Texas, Central America, and the West Indies. The latter part of the botanical name, *aphrodisiaca*, indicates the herb's reputed value for arousing sexual desire.

Early Uses

In the 1900s, Dr. W. H. Meyers, an American physician, reported that he had given Mexican damiana an extensive trial in his practice and found that "in cases of partial impotence and sexual debility, its success is universal."

The herb was also cited as an effective remedy for impotence in other medical writings which appeared around the same time. Doctors Wood and Ruddock, for example, referred to damiana as having strong aphrodisiac power, adding that it use had cured "many cases of total or partial impotence where the usual remedies have given no relief." The recommended dosage was: "Of the fluid extract from 15 drops to a teaspoonful; of the solid extract three to six grains; of the sugar-coated pills, one or two."

Reported Modern Uses of Damiana

Mexican damiana is classed as aphrodisiac, stimulant, tonic, and diuretic. The herb has been scientifically accepted in Mexico as a reliable remedy for exhaustion, catarrhal inflammation of the bladder, and cases of sexual impotence especially when caused by excesses. It is also used for orchitis (inflammation of a testicle) and spermatorrhea (involuntary emissions). The plant is said to exert a favorable influence on the spinal column, and some Mexican physicians employ it as a brain tonic. It is also prescribed in nephritis (kidney inflammation).

In England and Germany, damiana is used for its aphrodisiac properties. In Holland, medical herbalist Steinmetz states that the herb is so esteemed not only for its sexual enhancing qualities, but also for "its excellent effect on the reproductive organs."

Instructions for Using Damiana

Mexican damiana may be used in the form of a tea or fluid extract. The tea is prepared with 1 teaspoon of the leaves to a cup of boiling water. The cup is covered with a saucer. The tea is allowed to steep (stand) for five minutes and is then strained. One cup is taken before breakfast and again later in the afternoon. Of the extract, Professor Martinez of Mexico suggests 50 drops (approx. 1 teaspoon) in a little sweetened water or wine taken daily before meals.

Combined Formula

The power of damiana as an aphrodisiac, or as a tonic for nervous or sexual debility, is said to increase when the leaves are combined with saw palmetto berries. Either of the following methods may be used:

Powdered Form Equal parts of powdered damiana leaves are mixed with equal parts of powdered saw palmetto berries. One to two teaspoons are taken each day in water or wine, or the powdered combination may be placed in gelatin capsules and swallowed with water.

Fluid Extracts One ounce each of the fluid extracts of damiana leaves and saw palmetto berries are mixed together, and 1 teaspoon is taken in a small glass of water three times daily before meals.

GRAVEL ROOT

Botanical Name: *Eupatorium purpureum*
Common Names: Joe-Pye Weed, Jopi Root, Kidney Root, Indian Root, Queen-of-the-Meadow

Gravel root is a purple flowered herb which grows on low, swampy grounds and can be seen skirting along moist banks. It is a native North American perennial with a rigidly erect stem usually about 5 or 6 feet high, though sometimes reaching higher.

Early Uses

Gravel root was a favorite remedy among various Indian tribes. Its common name of Joe-Pye (or Jopi) was given in honor of a New England Indian healer who used it to cure typhus by inducing profuse sweating. However, since one of its principal uses was for treating bladder and kidney complaints, the herb was commonly called gravel root and kidney root. Among the Cherokees and Iroquois, it was employed as a diuretic, while the Menomenees prepared decoctions of the root for urinary difficulties, gravel, and lower backache.

As with hundreds of other native herbal remedies, the use of gravel root was imparted by the Indians to the white settlers, who recognized its value as a healing agent quickly. The herb doctor H. B. Skinner considered a decoction of the root to be a strong diuretic which "removes strangury, gravel, and stone." Others reported its effectiveness in treating various bladder and kidney ailments.

Modern Uses The action of gravel root is classed as diuretic, stimulant, and tonic. The root is still widely employed by medical herbalists for eliminating gravel and stones from the kidneys and bladder. It is also used for water retention and to relieve lower back pain caused by kidney complaints

A decoction is prepared with 1 ounce of the root to 1-1/2 pints of boiling water. This is simmered slowly for half an hour and then strained. One-fourth of a cup is taken every three hours or as needed. If the tincture is used instead, it may be taken in doses of one teaspoonful in a small glass of water.

AGNUS CASTUS

Botanical Name: *Vitex agnus castus*
Common Names: Chaste Tree, Nunswort, Chaste Bush

For many years agnus castus has been used by the natives of the Balkans as a remedy for infertility. It is also recommended for the same purpose in England. For example, a distressed man contacted Dr. Bartram, explaining: "In spite of hospital tests my wife and I have been unable to conceive a child. They say there is no physical reason why I shouldn't have a child. . . What do you think?"

Dr. Bartram replied: "If you feel you cannot live without a child, there are many harmless herbs which have been successful in breaking down the barriers of infertility by promoting function of the ovaries and womb. One that springs to mind is agnus castus. Also known as nunswort, it exercises a powerful influence upon the womb and appears to have the property of normalizing hormone production to the point where conception is possible."

Agnus Castus for Male Disorders

Although agnus castus is credited with healing properties of special relevance to women, homeopaths have found the herb also to be effective in treating certain male disorders, especially the loss of sexual power. In homeopathy it is used in doses of the first to sixth potency for symptoms of impotence, genital parts cold and relaxed, desire gone; scanty emission without ejaculation; loss of prostatic fluid on straining to urinate, testicles cold, swollen, hard and painful.

UVA-URSI

Botanical Name: *Arctostaphylos uva-ursi*
Common Names: Bearberry, Kinnekinnick, Arberry

This small evergreen shrub is found growing on the hills and high mountains of America, Europe, and Asia. The leathery textured leaves are dark green on the surface but paler green on the lower side. They have no distinctive odor. The berries are bright red and glossy, consisting of a mealy pulp with an unpleasant taste.

Medicinal Uses

Uva-ursi is classed as astringent, diuretic, and tonic. The chief constituent of the leaves is a glucoside called *arbutin*. The dried leaves are the only part of the plant employed in herbal medicine, and the usual form of administration is that of an infusion. Uva-ursi is considered of great value in treating bladder and kidney complaints, strengthening and imparting tone to the urinary organs and to the mucous membrane of the whole urinary tract. It has a soothing as well as astringent effect, along with a pronounced diuretic action.

Medical herbalists explain that the diuretic action of uva-ursi comes from arbutin, which is largely absorbed unchanged and is excreted by the kidneys. During its excretion, arbutin produces an antiseptic effect of the urinary mucous membrane. An infusion of the leaves is therefore used in inflammatory diseases of the urinary tract, cystitis, urethritis, etc.

Uva-ursi tea is prepared by placing 1 ounce of the leaves in 1 pint of water. As soon as the water boils, the container is set aside and the tea is allowed to stand until cold and is then strained. One-half cupful is taken every four hours. If the tincture is used instead, 10 to 20 drops are taken in a small glass of water three or four times a day.

Uva-ursi for Incontinence

Incontinence is defined as the involuntary loss of bladder control. According to physicians, the major causes are inflammation of the urinary tract and the failure of the "signal system" caused by a variety of illnesses and medications. The use of alcohol can worsen the problem.

A retired pharmacist recommends the following for incontinence: "There is one simple remedy that has been found very useful in such cases. I hardly know how it operates, but it seems to be a tonic for the sphincter muscle of the bladder so as to prevent loss of bladder control. It is uva-ursi, half a teaspoonful of the powder in a cup of boiling water every morning."

Note. The use of uva-ursi sometimes colors the urine, but medical herbalists say there is no cause for concern.

SARSAPARILLA

Botanical Name: *Smilax officinalis*
Common Names: Honduras Sarsaparilla, Jamaica Sarsaparilla, Spanish Sarsaparilla

The name sarsaparilla is derived from two Spanish words, *sarza* (shrub) and *parilla* (little vine). The plant is a perennial, a genus of climbing or trailing vines or shrubs native to tropical America.

There are several varieties of commercial sarsaparilla (e.g., Honduras or brown sarsaparilla; Jamaica, Costa Rica, Central American, or red sarsaparilla; Vera Cruz, Mexican, or grey sarsaparilla). Authorities explain that care must be taken in choosing the commercial sarsaparilla since it may be of poor quality due to age or because it was obtained from an inferior species.

Early Uses

Sarsaparilla was well known to the Indians of Mexico and South America, who used it for treating sexual impotence, rheumatism, skin ailments, and as a tonic for physical weakness.

Gerard, and early English herbalist, speaks of "Zarsaparilla of Peru" sent over from "countries of the New World called America." He recommends it for continual aches and pains in the joints and "against cold diseases." News of the plant medicine gradually spread to many other parts of the world. Old-time drug stores carried a wide variety of sarsaparilla preparations, and writings on the virtues of the plant and could be found in medical journals, newspapers, magazines, and almanacs. It was cited as a spring tonic and as a remedy for a long list of ailments including syphilis, sexual impotence, gout, chronic rheumatism, digestive disorders, and skin problems.

The popularity of sarsaparilla continued until the late nineteenth century, but then it fell into disuse when its medicinal benefits were considered to be only superstitious ignorance. At that point it would have faded into oblivion had it not been that the plant was found to contain valuable properties as a base for compound syrups. Later, after an in-depth review of more recent evidence, Perutz (*Handb. d Haut-und Geschlechtesdrank*, 1928.) concluded that sarsaparilla does have some remedial value, probably by stimulating the body's defense system. Then in 1931 Philippsohn (*Derm. Wchnschr.*, 1931, 93, 1220) cited the use of an extract of sarsaparilla in cases of psoriasis. Other medical findings on the beneficial effects of the plant for this troublesome skin disorder were also reported by Grutz and Bürger, (*Klin. Wchnschr.*, 1933), Ritter, (*Deutsche med. Wchnschr.*, 1936) and Thurmon (*New Eng. J. Med.*, 1942).

Further Research

In the U.S. a search for hormones, or what may be called prohormones in botanical substances, was undertaken by Professor Russell E. Marker and Dr. Ewald Rohrmon of Pennsylvania State College. Hundreds of plants were tested, but it was not until they began to experiment with an extract of sarsaparilla roots that they were successful.

The first hormone found by Marker and Rohrmon was testosterone, but the medical profession paid little attention to their announcement of this important fact. It was not until later when the *New York Times* (Aug. 11, 1946) reported the story of a discovery in Mexico of testosterone in sarsaparilla that sufficient notice was given to the matter.

Progesterone and cortin are two other hormones that have been found in the root of the plant.

The discoveries in America and Mexico were apparently made independently of each other. A Hungarian scientist, Dr. Emerick Solomo, had lived in Mexico for some years and was curious about a remedy used by the Indians as a cure for sexual impotence, physical debility, and weakness. He decided to investigate the merits of the remedy and conducted exhaustive tests with sarsaparilla root. His findings were the same as those of Marker and Rohrmon. Dr. Solomo conducted thousands of tests on animals and men which established conclusively that sarsaparilla hormones do benefit their users.

How Sarsaparilla Is Used

Sarsaparilla is classed as alterative, tonic, and diaphoretic. It may be given in the form of a decoction made with 1 ounce of the root boiled slowly in 1-1/2 pints of water for 20 minutes. The strained decoction is taken frequently in wineglassful doses.

Sarsaparilla is also available on the market in the form of tablets, fluid extracts, and the powdered root contained in gelatin capsules.

SUMMARY

1. Time-tested herbs can help relieve a variety of genito-urinary problems.

2. Certain herbs produce good results when used alone but in some cases may be employed to greater advantage when combined with other botanicals.

3. Buchu tea should never be allowed to boil continuously, as this would destroy the plant's essential oils responsible for its antiseptic and antibacterial action.

4. Although the herb agnus castus is credited with healing properties of special relevance to women, homeopathic doctors have found it to be effective in treating male disorders as well.

5. The use of uva-ursi sometimes colors the urine, but according to medical herbalists there is no cause for concern.

6. Researchers have discovered that sarsaparilla contains the hormones testosterone, progesterone, and cortin.

ENDNOTES

1. *Health from Herbs,* Jan.-Feb. 1969.

2. *Health from Herbs,* Jan.-Feb. 1969.

3. *Nature's Healing Agents* (Quakertown, PA: The Humanitarian Society Reg.), 1960.

4. C. J. Bishop and R. E. MacDonald, *Canadian Journal of Botany,* 1951.

5. *Grace,* Winter 1968.

6. *Health from Herbs,* Sept.-Oct. 1968.

C H A P T E R   6

HERB REMEDIES FOR OBSTINATE ULCERS, BURNS, AND WOUNDS

Nature has provided a large variety of herbs and herbal substances for coping with these painful disorders. Since it is not possible to cover all of them in one chapter, only the most common examples are presented here.

COMFREY

Botanical Name: *Symphytum officinale*
Common Names: Knitbone, Bruisewort, Woundwort

Comfrey is native to Europe and temperate Asia but is naturalized in the United States, growing on low grounds and country lanes. It is a perennial with large, hairy, prickly leaves and bears whitish pale-purple flowers. The spindle-shaped root spreads in thick branches underground and penetrates deeply into the earth.

The common names of knitbone, bruisewort, and woundwort indicate its use from earliest times as a remedy for treating injuries. It was also used for ulcers, bed sores, growths, and skin irritations.

Early Medical Use

Charles J. Macalister, M.D., first learned of comfrey's healing power in 1911 and decided to use the herb in his medical practice. The results he achieved and the subsequent chemical analysis proved that comfrey contains a valuable healing agent called *allantoin*, a cell proliferant found in the leaves and roots.

Dr. Macalister cited several cases in which comfrey, or allantoin derived from comfrey was used.[1] About a 48-year-old woman whose case was transferred to his care, he wrote:

> There was a large ulcer on the dorsum of the foot and another practically continuous with it over the lower third of the leg. The bases were in places sloughy and even gangrenous looking, and there was a purulent discharge. She was sent to Dr. Crawford, I understood, for his opinion as to whether the leg should be amputated. The ulcer measured five inches by four inches, and had been in existence for five years. Allantoin dressings were commenced on July 25th. A week later the surface had cleaned and presented healthy granulations, and a rapid growth of epitheleum was taking place from all the margins. On August 12th it was manifestly healing, and on August 17th, i.e. in 23 days, this huge ulcer was reduced to the size of a pin's head. The scar was healthy and sound. The patient was kept in bed for a fortnight (two weeks), and after her discharge it remained sound and well.

Dr. Macalister also mentions the results obtained by other physicians who were treating their patients with comfrey. For example, an 83-year-old man was seen by Dr. Charles Searle of Cambridge on October 23, 1911. For some months the patient's condition was considered grave, as he had marked arteriosclerosis, low temperature, feeble pulse, and a loud "aortic systolic murmur." Dr. Searle reported:

> During December 1911, a fungating ulcer appeared on the dorsum of the left foot. It rapidly spread, and eventually exposed the metatarsal bones. In January, 1912, the patient's condition appeared to be hopeless, he became at times delirious, and was removed home to die. He was then treated with four-hourly fomentations made with decoction of Comfrey root. The ulcer immediately began to fill up rapidly and was practically healed by the end of April, and the patient's condition made corresponding improvement.

Modern Medical Uses

In his book *Nature's Healing Grasses*[2], Dr. H. E. Kirschner, M.D., devotes four chapters to the subject of comfrey. It is apparent from his writings on the subject that his experiences with the medicinal use of the herb substantiate the findings of Dr. Macalister and other early physicians. For example, he tells of a woman who was troubled by a nipple-shaped growth on the side of her nose which was treated by her doctor in the usual orthodox manner. But the curative effects of the treatment were only temporary, and before long the growth returned.

The woman's son, deeply concerned about his mother's condition and having read articles written by Dr. Kirschner on the miracle working properties of comfrey, suggested that perhaps a comfrey root poultice might relieve the fast-growing wart. His mother agreed to give the remedy a try, so the next day Dr. Kirschner shipped a bottle of comfrey root powder to her.

Dr. Kirschner writes: "Small poultices were immediately applied to her nose during the daytime and a large poultice was worn at night. Almost immediately the inflamed condition subsided, and the nasty growth began to recede. The recession was slow but gradual, and in less than 60 days the once ugly 'wart' had completely disappeared. Today even close examination fails to show a trace of this once distressing growth, and there are no tell-tale scars."

Dr. Alfred Vogel of Switzerland also considers comfrey to be a valuable healing agent.[3] He says it has been successfully used for "suppurating ulcers, wounds which refuse to heal, and leg ulcers." He adds, "there is hardly a better remedy to be found for the external treatment of gout; the raw root should be finely grated and applied to the affected parts like a poultice. If the fresh roots are not available, the tincture can be used instead. The latter is also very effective in *neuralgic* pains, especially facial *neuralgia*."

Comfrey as a Home Remedy

The following recent case studies show the various ways in which comfrey has been used and the conditions it has remedied.

"My grandson injured his toenail. The doctor operated, removing the half of it where it attached to the toe. After one year it was still sore, exuding pus and lymph. My grandson and his mother visited me, and I felt that comfrey poultices might help. After three weeks a 1/2-inch by 1/16-inch piece of toenail showed up. In another week it was well and hasn't troubled him since—more than a year now." —Mrs. A. McL.

"When my 85-year-old mother-in-law became ill and bedridden, she developed an angry-looking bed sore. Months of medical treatments did not help, so my husband and I began searching through a number of health books and came across one which recommended comfrey for bed sores.

"According to instructions, we prepared a comfrey root decoction. After it was carefully strained and cooled to just barely warm, we filled an ear syringe with the liquid and syringed the sore several times. Then we made up a poultice by stirring powdered comfrey root in water to make a paste. We smeared the mixture inside a small cloth bag and applied it to the bed sore, changing my mother-in-law's position to keep her off the painful area.

"The entire treatment was repeated three times every day. In about two weeks, we noticed granulations forming around the edges of the sore. As time passed the bed sore began getting smaller, and in about two-and-a-half months it was completely healed." —M. W. L.

"I feel I must and tell you how I overcame a badly sprained ankle. I was running to catch a train when I twisted my ankle. At first it didn't hurt much, but by the time I arrived home it had swollen twice its normal size and was very painful. As the evening wore on it became worse. Then I remembered comfrey and how good it is for sprains and bruises, so I applied a few leaves in a cold water compress around my ankle. The result was astounding. After roughly one-and-a-half hours the pain had lessened considerably, and I was able to walk with ease. Next morning, although the ankle was still swollen, there was no pain and I was able to get to work." —Mrs. J. C.

"An intricate dental operation lasting an hour left me with one side of my face hugely swollen. Since I live in the country where comfrey plants grow in abundance in the lanes, I picked some leaves, stirred them in water and then used the leaves and water to make a poultice. I slipped it on my face, and inside the hour the swelling had gone down dramatically. A few more applications and it had almost vanished." —Mr. H. B.

A medical herbalist writes: "What a good friend we have in comfrey! A few days ago I hurt my foot and could hardly walk for the pain and swelling. We have scores of efficient remedies on our shelves but the one I selected was comfrey. I made a simple infusion of boiling water and dried comfrey leaves and gave my foot a good bathing. This happened during the week; by Saturday I was back at the Consulting Rooms with it almost completely better. You can even use an infusion to bathe swollen joints in rheumatism, and bruises." —L. M., M.N.I.M.H.[4] Member of the National Institute of Medical Herbalists.

HONEY

The value of honey as a food and curative agent has been known for thousands of years. It is frequently mentioned in the Bible. Miriam administered it to the baby Moses on the river Nile by anointing him with "a finger of honey to save him from the ravages of sunshine." The sacred books of Persia, Egypt, India, China, and others also refer to the healing power of honey. The Koran speaks of it as an excellent medicine and wholesome food. Mohammed proclaimed, "Honey is a remedy for all diseases."

The Egyptian papyri cited the value of honey not only as a food but especially as a medicine. It was used internally for many ailments and externally in medical dressings for ulcers, burns, and skin diseases.

The Greek physician Hippocrates treated a variety of illnesses with honey, claiming that is also "cleans sores and ulcers, softens hard ulcers of the lips, heals carbuncles and running sores."

Modern Medical Uses of Honey

Several British hospitals reportedly use honey for scalds, burns, and ulcers. For example, Dr. Robert Blomfield states: "I have been using pure natural honey in the accident and emergency departments where I work." He explains that he applies honey under a dry dressing every two or three days and has found that "it promotes healing of ulcers and burns better than any other local application I've used before."

Reported Uses of Honey as a Home Remedy

People from all parts of the world have found that many painful conditions respond exceptionally well to the magic touch of honey. One man reported that his wife sustained a severe burn about 4 inches in length on her wrist.

He immediately applied a thick coating of honey to the affected area and covered it with a bandage. Within 10 minutes she was free from pain. After 20 hours the bandage was removed, and her husband exclaimed, "You can imagine our surprise to find no sign of blistering or damage to the skin. This might help other readers should they be faced with a similar situation."

Mrs. A. O. tells of her experience with the use of honey. She says she developed a huge lump at the base of her spine. Her doctor informed her it was a large abscess which would require many weeks of treatment. Mrs. O. was instructed not to return to work and to apply "poultices of epsom salts to the abscess every two or three hours daily." She says, "It was going to be a horrible few weeks ahead: I was told there would be a big hole left where the swelling had been."

Following the doctor's instructions, she proceeded with the applications, and as one head appeared on the abscess the doctor lanced it. Soon another head started to form, and by this time the surrounding skin was getting extremely tender. Mrs. O. then decided to discontinue the medical treatment and try honey instead. She writes: "I spread the abscess liberally with honey and lots of talc; plus a dressing of course. Within two weeks it had shriveled down to a small lump. No more heads formed and no more discomfort. After a very short space of time, it completely disappeared. I have no mark at all to show where the abscess was!"

Another remarkable case is that of a woman who was deep-frying some food in her kitchen using a small iron saucepan. When finished, she poured the boiling oil into a white basin. Turning around to clean the saucepan, and without thinking, she accidentally grabbed the hot basin of oil. Dropping it with a gasp, some of the boiling oil splashed over the palm of her hand. She says: "I was in agony. Being alone, I was frantic. Then my attention was turned to a jar of honey on the table. I placed a large teaspoonful of honey into my palm and dressed it awkwardly as best I could with a bandage. Believe it or not, the next morning I could once more move my fingers. After another day the improvement was amazing. No evidence of the injury could be seen except for skinned skin between the fingers. All the pain had gone out of it!"

Mrs. C. H. tells of how she found honey to be an effective remedy for boils. She writes: "My late husband had boils on his neck, as he carried cement bags at his work. Nothing seemed to help. An old lady told me to get flour and honey, mix a paste, spread it on a piece of white paper, stick it on the boil, and leave it on until it came off. When I took it off, there was a long root leaving a wee hole. No more boils after that."

Mrs. M. R. also pays tribute to the healing power of honey. She reports that her husband suffered a nasty accident at cricket—his finger was badly split. She explains: "It was bandaged up, and when I saw the finger later at home, I didn't know how to treat it. We went to a health food store I know of, and the assistant there advised us to apply liquid honey on a piece of bandage two or three times daily on the wound, saying that the wound would heal perfectly without leaving a scar. We did this, and after the second application the finger was eased and cleansed, and in three weeks the wound was healed perfectly, the flesh knitting together without even a scar. What a wonderful thing!"

F. T. tells of leg ulcers effectively treated with honey: "A friend had dreadful ulcers on her leg for years. A few months ago she was having them medically dressed twice a week. Mother and I begged her to dress them with honey, and take it internally. Of course, she was afraid to do so. But at last she plucked up courage. Within days those awful scabs had crumbled and her leg healed wonderfully."

The following report appeared in an early edition of *Alpenlandishe Bienenzeitung* (Feb. 1935): "In the winter of 1935 I heated a boiler of about thirty-five gallons of water. When I opened the cover, it flew with great force against the ceiling. The vapor and hot water poured forth over my unprotected head, over my hands and feet. Some minutes afterward I had violent pains and I believe I would have gone mad it my wife and daughter had not helped me immediately. They took large pieces of linen, daubed them thickly with honey and put them on my head, neck, hands, and feet. Almost instantly the pain ceased. I slept well all night and did not lose a single hair on my head. When the physician came, he shook his head and said, 'How can such a thing be possible?'"

ST. JOHN'S WORT

Botanical Name: *Hypericum perforatum*
Common Name: Woundwort, Hypericum

St. John's Wort is a perennial herb growing from 2 to 3 feet high in meadows, fields, and on the banks of roadsides. The narrow, dark green leaves are dotted with small holes which can be seen when a leaf is held up to the light. Its flowers are bright yellow with many golden threads in the middle, and when bruised they yield a reddish juice.

There are many ancient superstitions regarding this herb. The name *Hypericum* shows that the plant was regarded as having magical powers over evil spirits. It is taken from two Greek words, *hyper* and *eikon* ("over" and "apparition"). In former times the herb was called Fuga Daemonum, or Scare-devil. On St. John's day, June 24, the plant was gathered and hung over the door or window, and in some lands it was worn as an amulet or charm.

Remedial Uses of St. John's Wort

Ages ago, herbalists such as Galen, Dioscorides, and Culpeper recommended St. John's Wort as an effective remedy for wounds and bruises. Modern practitioners of natural healing methods have found that these early herbalists were correct. St. John's Wort is a specific for lacerated wounds and for painful injuries to the nerves and areas richly supplies with nerves, such as the spine, fingers, and toes. For example, from years of treating patients with the herbal remedy, Dr. Dorothy Shepherd reports:[5] "I much prefer Hypericum (St. John's Wort) tincture, applied locally, to any of the modern antiseptics; it does not destroy the healthy tissues and healthy cells; it cleans up dirty, septic wounds; it eases the inflammation in septic fingers, in boils, in cellulitis and lymphangitis. Lacerated, crushed fingers and hands remain surgically clean and aseptic, and heal rapidly in consequence."

Dr. Shepherd cites the case of a woman who slipped and fell, landing on her coccyx (tail bone). She suffered excruciating pains radiating up her spine. The patient was given homeopathic tablets of St. John's Wort in the thirtieth potency every two hours, then every four hours, and then three times daily, which "cured her completely in a few days without hindering her in her daily work at all."

ECHINACEA

Botanical Name: *Echinacea angustifolia*
Common Names: Coneflower, Purple Coneflower

Practitioners of natural medicine explain that boils, abscesses, and carbuncles result from a disordered condition of the bloodstream. To correct this condition, the herb echinacea, classed as a blood purifier, is the remedy most often recommended. For example, in his book *Nature's Healing Agents*, Dr. Swinburne Clymer writes: "Irrespective of all that has been said, written and printed about Echinacea, the true Physio-Medicalist has found it to be the one supreme and dependable remedy to combat morbidity of the blood."[6] He recommends its use for cellular abscesses, carbuncles, and toxemia.

Dr. W. H. Felter, a former therapeutic editor of the *American Dispensatory*[7], also regarded echinacea as a natural blood antitoxin. He reported: "Echinacea is a remedy for autointoxication, and whenever the blood stream becomes slowly infected either from within or without the body. Elimination is imperfect, the body tissues become altered and there is developed within the fluids and tissues septic action with adynamia, resulting in boils, carbuncles, cellular tissue inflammations, abscesses and other systemic processes."

Potter's Encyclopedia of Botanical Drugs and Preparations[8] cites the value of echinacea as "useful in all diseases due to impurities in the blood, such as boils, carbuncles, gangrene, etc., internally and externally."

How Echinacea Is Used

When the *standard extract* of echinacea is employed, one-half to one teaspoon is taken in a small glass of water three to four times a day. If using the *standard tincture*, 15 to 30 drops in a small glass of water may be taken every one to three hours as necessary.

A *homeopathic tincture* of echinacea is also available and can be obtained from homeopathic pharmacies, health food stores, and herb firms. For adults, 25 drops of the tincture are stirred in one-half glass of water. Two teaspoons of the mixture are taken every one or two hours in acute affections, and every three or four hours in lesser affections (one-half teaspoon of the mixture for children).

Note. Either of the tinctures or extracts may also be applied directly to the boil, abscess or carbuncle.

Case Study

An interesting letter comes from Mr. W. P. of Stoke-on-Kent, who says, "I read an article about echinacea and treated my friend with it for persistant boils, giving him 10 drops of the extract in water at a time. He only had to take a total of three to four ounces and he hasn't had a boil since."

MARIGOLD

Botanical Name: *Calendula officinalis*
Common Name: Calendula, Pot Marigold, Holigold

The common marigold is a well-known garden plant with its pale green leaves and golden-orange flowers. Its generic name *calendula* means "flower of the calends," and in some areas it is in bloom throughout the year. In former times, marigold flowers were dried for broths and soups and used to add color to salads and cheeses.

During World War I, homeopathic physicians of the Allied Forces discovered that a solution of marigold had a remarkable healing effect on the wounds of injured soldiers in septic states of the tissues. German medics made the same discovery. The solution proved especially effective for lacerated wounds and suppurations. To this day, homeopaths consider marigold to be one of the best antiseptics, and it seems likely that the herb's power is due to its content of natural iodine.

Modern Remedial Uses of Marigold

As a remedy, marigold is often used in various forms such as tinctures, ointments, or creams. Herbalists regard these preparations effective for cuts, sprains, bruises, and ulcerations. They are also reputed to be of special value for severe burns, promoting healing and often preventing the formation of scar tissue. Combined with vinegar, the tincture is said to be an effective wash to reduce and strengthen varicose veins.

In reference to the use of marigold, Dr. Eric Powell writes:[9]

> An infusion of the dried petals may be used, but the best results are obtained by using either compresses of the fully gathered petals, or from the fresh plant tincture distilled with water, which should be hot for preference. Up to an ounce (of the tincture) to a pint of hot water may be used for this purpose. Boils and nasty skin eruptions respond promptly to the healing effects.

Case Studies

"I felt I must tell you what a wonderful success marigold cream is. I had a very nasty gash on my arm. I was passing through an open door with my arms loaded, when the wind caught it and the tongue of the new lock caught my arm. It was as if the flesh had been sliced with a knife. Of course, it bled. To staunch the bleeding I put on clean lint. Then I suddenly thought of marigold, to use especially if the skin is broken. I smothered the wound with the cream, covering it up with a large plaster, and left it completely alone for four days. There was no pain or soreness. When I had a look I could scarcely believe my eyes. It was practically healed. It was absolutely wonderful." —Mrs. G. M.

"Calendula is a fantastic healer—not only the ointment but the tincture also. Place six drops tincture calendula in a tablespoon of warm water. Apply to any open wound, cut, or laceration, and the bleeding will stop at once. Bind it up. In a few days the chances are it will have cleared. This tincture has been an alternative to the stitching up of injured skin over and over again. I am never without it in the house." —Mrs. H. L. D.

"Perhaps this simple remedy may help someone else. I had a nasty cracked lip which wouldn't heal (even after using my favorite castor oil). Two days after applying calendula cream, it was back to normal." —J. H.

CASTOR OIL PLANT

Botanical Name: *Ricinus communis*
Common Name: Palma Christi

The castor oil plant is cultivated in many temperate regions throughout the world as a stately annual and for its seeds, from which a fixed oil is expressed. When fully expanded, its handsome, palmately lobed leaves are of a blue-green color, but when young they are red and shiny. The plant bears male and female flowers on clustered, oblong spikes.

Reported External Uses of Castor Oil

When used externally, castor oil has an impressive record as a healing agent for many troublesome conditions:

"My late sister, some years ago, was suffering from a rather nasty varicose ulcer while living overseas. The leg had been responding slowly to a mud pack which originated from a famous Austrian resort.

"The treatment came to an end before the ulcer had completely healed, when the mud ran out. Fresh supplies were difficult to acquire, as we were living in sanctions-ridden Rhodesia at the time.

"My sister had been reading that castor oil might help. She began daily applications of the remedy. The result after only a few days astounded her. Quite soon the ulcer was completely healed." —Mrs. S. S.

"I had a papilloma on my eyelid which had been there for about six months. Having heard of the benefits of castor oil when applied to warts and corns, I thought I'd try it on the papilloma. For one or two minutes, three times a day, I rubbed the oil on it, gently but thoroughly. The papilloma began to grow smaller, and in four weeks it was gone.

"My brother, who had a papilloma near the side of his nose which had been there for some years, was so impressed with my results he decided to try the oil for himself. In three months there was no longer any trace of the papilloma." —Mrs. R. T.

"About 30 years ago I had a nasty varicose ulcer. Some months later, as it was still as bad, a different doctor told me to keep off my legs as much as possible for two months. I was to lie on a sofa all day and bandage the ulcer with castor oil liniment, morning and evening. It worked wonders. It left a large brown scar, which gradually disappeared. I am 94 years old and feeling fit and well." —Mrs. I. M. E.

"I had a broken chilblain on my big toe which became an ulcer and was septic. I had months under a doctor's care, having antibiotics, etc. I tried honey, which kept it clean, but it still did not heal.

"Then in an old copy of *Grace* I read about castor oil for healing. I applied this; in three days it started to heal. Soon it was completely better. Last week I cut my leg and it left a nasty wet place, so I applied castor oil. It healed immediately. I am over 70 and must be careful with leg injuries, so I am very grateful for all this help." —E. H.

ALOE VERA

Botanical Name: *Aloe vera*
Common Names: Barbados Aloe, Medicine Plant, Lily of the Desert

This tropical plant is native to South Africa, Europe, and other countries bordering the Mediterranean but it has spread to other suitable climates throughout the world. In appearance it is similar to some forms of cacti; however, it is not a cactus but a member of the lilacea family, which includes lilies and onions. Its fleshy speckled green leaves are about 2 feet long, spear-like, and edged with spiny teeth. From the center of the plant a long stalk rises which bears a dense cluster of yellow and red tubular blossoms. When the inner part of the leaf is cut, it secretes a clear gel which contains healing properties.

Medicinal Uses

Aloe gel is used for sunburn, thermal burns, radiation burns, and other different burns of all kinds. It seems to have the remarkable power of regenerating the skin and damaged tissues. In the treatment of burns it quickly relieves pain, reduces inflammation, and prevents blistering. Little or no scar tissue is formed.

The gel is also used to treat wounds, bed sores, ulcers, erysipelas, ring worm, shingles, poison oak, poison ivy, and many other complaints. When applied to a small cut it immediately arrests bleeding, as it dries very rapidly. Applied to the exposed areas of the body, the gel acts as an insect repellent. It also treats skin blemishes, acne, and pimples.

Methods of Using Aloe Vera

The gel from a potted, mature aloe plant can be obtained by slicing the inner part of one of the leaves with a knife. However, it is not necessary to grow an aloe plant to take advantage of its healing properties. Many health food stores and herb firms carry numerous products which utilize aloe gel as an important ingredient. Some authorities caution, however, that unless any brand of aloe vera ointment or cream contains at least 70% of aloe concentration, it won't be of much benefit. Cosmetic products such as skin fresheners, moisturizers, facial gels, and cleansers should contain at least 40% of aloe vera concentration. Percentages are usually listed on the labels of the products.

Case Studies Show Aloe Offers Impressive Results

A news article on aloe vera[10] reported the case of a 22-year-old woman who suffered from a form of psoriasis. According to the article, her doctor prescribed a medicated salve which proved ineffective. The woman then decided to try aloe vera, which she grew as a potted plant in her home. She was amazed when the itching of her troublesome skin condition stopped immediately after the first application of aloe gel.

The same article also cited the case of a young man who suffered for months from a severe case of painful hemorrhoids, for which surgery was required. Three years after surgery the problem returned, and he was faced with another operation. Recalling the excruciating pain, he rebelled at the idea of more surgery. But the following year, the hemorrhoidal pain was so intense he could no longer work or even move about normally. He then heard about aloe vera from a relative and decided to try rectal applications of the gel in the form of a homemade suppository. Within one week, the pain completely vanished.

Karen Gottleib, Ph.D., reports a number of cases effectively treated with aloe vera.[11] In one case a man had suffered from varicose ulcers of the leg for 15 years. The two large ulcers were described as "deep and foul-smelling." He was medically treated with a special preparation of stabilized aloe vera pulp by doctors in Cairo, Egypt. After one week the ulcers began to heal. Regeneration of the skin was evident after four weeks. Two weeks later the upper part of the larger ulcer was much smaller, and the lower half was completely healed.

Another case Gottlieb reports concerns that of a man who worked in a canning factory and accidentally stepped into a vat of boiling water up to his knees. "His burns were so serious that the layer of skin came off with his clothes. Holes the size of silver dollars were burned through to the inner layer of his skin."

The patient was treated by Dr. J. E. Crewe of Minnesota, who prepared a special ointment consisting of an equal amount of powdered aloes and mineral oil in a vaseline base. The preparation was spread on sterile gauze and wrapped around the patient's legs. Incredibly, the pain was kept at a minimum level and there was no sign of infection. The healing took place rapidly and without formation of scar tissue. After just 10 days the raw areas could no longer be seen, and within three weeks of the accident the man was able to return to work.

SUMMARY

1. Comfrey contains allantoin, a cell proliferant which accounts for the herb's remarkable healing power in treating conditions of wounds, ulcers, bed sores, warts, etc.

2. Burns and many other painful conditions have responded exceptionally well when treated with honey.

3. Tincture of St. John's Wort is a specific for lacerated wounds and injuries to the nerves and areas richly supplied with nerves (e.g., spine, fingers, and toes).

4. Echinacea, classed as a blood purifier, is considered effective in treating certain problems resulting rom a disordered condition of the blood. Abscesses, boils, and carbuncles are some examples.

5. Marigold ointment, tincture, or cream is used for cuts, sprains, bruises, and ulcerations.

6. When applied topically, castor oil has an impressive record as a healing agent for many troublesome conditions.

7. The gel of aloe vera is used for different burns of all kinds and also treats many other complaints.

8. According to some authorities, any brand of aloe vera ointment or cream should contain at least 70% of aloe concentration; cosmetic products should contain at least 40%.

ENDNOTES

1. *Narrative of an Investigation Concerning an Ancient Medicinal Remedy and Its Modern Utilities* (Lee Foundation for Nutritional Research: Milwaukee, WI), 1962.

2. Copyright by Anna Louise White. (Riverside, CA: H. C. White Publications, 1960), p. 60.

3. *The Nature Doctor* (Teufen(AR) Switzerland: Bioforce-Verlag) 7th edition.

4. *Health from Herbs*, July 1957.

5. *A Physicians' Posy* (Rustington, Sussex, England: Health Science Press, 1969).

6. Quakertown, PA: The Humanitarian Society, Reg., 1960.

7. H. W. Felter, M.D., *Echinacea* (Cincinnati, OH: Lloyd Bros., Inc., n.d.).

8. F. L. S. Wren (London: Sir Isaac Pitman & Sons, Ltd., 1956).

9. *Fitness and Health from Herbs*, May 1963.

10. Paul Reining, *Nat'l. Tattler*, 1973.

11. *Aloe Vera Heals* (Denver, CO: Royal Publications, Inc., 1984).

CHAPTER 7

HERBS FOR GASTROINTESTINAL AND BOWEL COMPLAINTS

In former times, almost every home had its own herb garden, and Grandma seemed to know just which herb was best to settle the stomach and which one would deal effectively with bowel troubles or intestinal complaints. These natural remedies are still with us today and are rapidly regaining their former popularity as effective healers. Consider the following examples:

"Ever since I was a child I had trouble with diarrhea, with many bouts of colitis, and with ulcerative colitis (on and off for about two years). I had all kinds of tests and X-rays, but they could not find any cause. They simply told me I would have to learn to live with it for the rest of my life, but I had no intention of doing so. You've got to do something for yourself if you want to get well.

"I felt sure there was an herb for every complaint, so I began taking Fenulin, a preparation of fenugreek seeds, and am delighted that the bowels are now normal." —Mrs. V. C.

"I have found calamus root tablets very helpful for my condition. After having tried to find something to give relief to my spastic colon for so long, calamus has helped me enormously." —Mr. T. R.

"My husband was bothered with constipation for years and had to rely on pills until a friend told him to take a tablespoon of crude blackstrap molasses in the morning and at night when retiring. It has done the job, and he doesn't need the pills now." —Mrs. G. A.

"One of the best remedies I know for piles is dandelion root, burdock, and yellow dock root. My mother had been bothered with piles for years and sometimes had to stay in because they were so bad. She drank a liquid mixture of the three herbs daily for about three months and never ever was bothered with piles again." —J. R. M.

"I am so happy since I found out about papaya tablets. I was always filled with gas—even water caused gas. This has disappeared like magic since taking the tablets." —Mrs. R. V.

"My daughter was greatly relieved of acid indigestion accompanied by terrible sour eructations after I gave her a tea made from calamus root. It has also benefitted me greatly, and I recommend it to everyone." —J. T.

"I thought you would be interested in the healing I have just experienced. Since May I have been under the care of a specialist for severe indigestion and looseness of the bowels. After a barium X-ray and barium enema, it was decided to give me an internal examination under anesthetic , as the specialist found an abnormality on the X-ray plate.

"In the meantime, six months altogether, I started taking Slippery Elm—a favorite remedy with my mother. I took the herb tablets twice a day and a good drink of the herb powder with milk as a nightcap.

"At the final examination the specialist seemed quite baffled. He sat on the bed and said 'There had been something there, but now there is only a little inflammation and we'll leave it to heal naturally.' With God's blessings, I know I have been healed." —E. E. of Cambridgeshire[1]

Just because a healing method is old does not mean that it is useless. Even medical herbalists of the Space Age still effectively treat their patients with the same herbs as did their earlier counterparts, but of course with the added advantage of modern research and technology.

HERBS: NATURE'S HEALING AGENTS

The herbs discussed in this chapter are examples of standard natural remedies which have remained consistent over the ages.

FENUGREEK

Botanical Name: *Trigonella foenum-graecum*
Common Names: Greek Hay-Seed, Bird's Food

Fenugreek is a leguminous herb, about 1 or 2 feet high with sickle-shaped pods, each consisting of from 10 to 20 edible mucilaginous seeds. The name of the genus, *Trigonella*, is taken from an old Greek name meaning "three-angled," from the shape of the herb's corolla. The plant is native to the eastern shores of the Mediterranean but has been cultivated in many other parts of the world.

Powdered fenugreek seed is used as a maple flavoring in confectionery. It is also an important ingredient in chutney, and in Oriental curry recipes for lamb, etc. In some countries the seeds are roasted and brewed as a substitute for coffee. They have also been employed for medicinal purposes since earliest of times.

Remedial Uses of Fenugreek

Fenugreek is classed as demulcent, nutritive, carminative, emollient, and expectorant. It is used internally as a tea for inflamed conditions of the stomach, bowels, and intestines.

Fenugreek is also one of the finest of all herbal aids for cleansing the body fouled by excessive mucus and slime, a condition caused by years of poor diet plus the long-standing habit of eating very large quantities of dairy products and other albuminous foods.

Not all the mucus from the throat, nose, and lungs is completely coughed up. Some of it enters the stomach and continues on to the kidneys and intestines. where it accumulates and hardens. When the stomach and intestines are saturated with mucus and slime, they cannot do an adequate job of discharging waste fluids.

As the thick, ropey mucus continues to build, the lining of the stomach, intestines, and bowels becomes irritated or inflamed. Distresses such as gas pains, diverticulitis, indigestion, halitosis, colitis, constipation, and other problems can then occur.

Methods of Using Fenugreek

A beverage of fenugreek seeds softens and dissolves hardened masses of mucus and produces a soothing, healing effect on inflamed areas. This ability is due to the mucilaginous consistency of the seeds from which the brew is made.

Fenugreek may be prepared in the stronger form of a decoction or in the milder form of an infusion (tea). The decoction is made by adding 2 teaspoons of the seeds to 1-1/2 cups of boiling water. This is simmered slowly for 10 minutes and then set aside and allowed to cool. One to three cups are taken daily.

The tea is prepared with 2 teaspoons of the seeds to 1 cup of water brought to a boil. As soon as the boiling point is reached, the vessel is removed from the burner and covered with a lid. The tea is allowed to stand for 15 minutes, and one cup is taken twice daily.

Fenugreek is also available in tablet form, with directions for use on the bottle.

Fenugreek for Diverticulosis

Dr. Bartram writes:[2]

Diverticulosis (known as diverticulitis when the site is inflamed) is a condition marked by the formation of small pouches along the border of the colon. These may become filled with feces, setting up chronic irritation. Abscesses may follow.

A remedy of proven ability in this field is fenugreek. Time and time again it proves supportive for toning smooth muscle tissue and for dispelling pain.

Dr. Bartram suggest drinking one, two, or three cupfuls of the *decoction* (including ingestion of the seeds) daily. He adds, "While fenugreek cannot do the impossible, it has brought peace and quiet to an otherwise angry bowel."

Case Studies

"My husband is so grateful for fenugreek. He won't be without it. It has made such a difference to his life. He was permanently on prescription drugs. He is now free from mucous colitis most of the time. When he does get pain, it only lasts a couple of days." —M. L.

"I used fenugreek tablets for my diverticulitis, which I have had for over two years. The doctor's treatment was disappointing, yet fenugreek gave remarkable improvement. I also feel so much better in myself. I can now go out all day without any trouble. I am 81 years old, and it is a great relief to feel so good." —Mrs. M. E.

"As I have diverticulitis, I have been taking fenugreek tablets, which I find very helpful." —Mrs. M. E.

"I have done so well on fenugreek tea for my colitis condition that I told a friend to try it after hospital tests showed she had diverticulitis. She is using the tea and getting excellent results." —Mrs. A. T.

"I am 71 years old and have suffered with colitis for 12 months. Having been unsuccessfully treated at a hospital for a year, taking up to seven different medicines at one time, I decided to try a natural remedy.

"I went to my health food shop and they recommended Fenulin tablets (a preparation of fenugreek seeds). I have been taking these for two weeks and am amazed at the results. It is the first time I have felt well for many months." —Miss S. A.[3]

PEPPERMINT

Botanical Name: *Mentha piperita*
Common Name: Brandy Mint

Peppermint is a perennial herb found in moist areas along streams and banks in all parts of Europe and the eastern U.S. It grows from 2 to 4 feet high, with dark green leaves smooth on the surface and finely toothed at the margins. The plant bears clusters of small, reddish-violet flowers, which appear from July to August.

Peppermint was first cultivated by the Egyptians thousands of years ago but is now commercially grown throughout the world.

Early Uses

The Romans crowned themselves with wreaths of peppermint at their banquets and decorated their tables with its sprays. They also used the herb freely in their food, not only for its flavor but also for its ability to expel gas from the stomach and bowels and to promote digestion. Roman women sweetened their breath with mint and honey after drinking wine.

In the New World, the Indians of the Missouri valley steeped the leaves of peppermint in water sweetened with sugar and drank the tea as a carminative. The Cheyennes ground the leaves and stems and boiled them as a decoction to prevent vomiting. Other tribes drank peppermint tea to relieve stomach distress and nausea. To break a fever, the tops and leaves of the plant were added to the sweat bath.

Among the early settlers, indigestion, gas cramps, bloating, and nausea were all treated with peppermint tea.

Modern Uses

Peppermint is classed as carminative, gastric stimulant, tonic, antiseptic, stomachic, and anodyne. A tea made from the leaves is still a popular beverage for coping with indigestion and resulting distresses. As a gastric stimulant, it tends to stimulate the flow of stomach digestive fluid so necessary to healthy digestion; as a stomachic and tonic it strengthens and tones the stomach; and as a carminative it helps to expel gas and relieve bloating. The age-old custom of serving mint sauce with spring lamb is no mere question of taste or fashion. All young meat is more difficult to digest than that of mature animals, and the addition of mint serves to prevent the meal from disagreeing.

Peppermint tea is prepared by placing a teaspoonful of the dried leaves in a cup and adding boiling water. The cup is covered with a saucer and allowed to stand for five minutes and is then strained. The infusion is drank in sips while very hot. (Reheat if necessary.)

A slight variation of the foregoing recipe of particular use when there are severe gas pains consists of mixing half a teaspoon of ground ginger with the mint leaves before adding the water.

Because of its action as a digestant, peppermint tea is best taken with meals.

Peppermint Oil Remedy for Irritable Bowel

Oil of peppermint has been found very helpful in conditions of irritable bowel syndrome (severe colicky abdominal cramps and distention). Herbalists suggest placing 2 drops of the oil in a coated empty gelatin capsule. One capsule is swallowed with a glass of water 10 minutes before meals three times daily. This enables the peppermint oil to be released slowly. By the time the capsule is dissolved, it is well past the stomach and duodenum and on its way through the intestines where its beneficial action is needed.

In conditions of irritable bowel, some attention should also be given to the diet. Examples of foods to be avoided include white bread, white sugar, salt, condiments, pickles, starchy and cream pastry, confectionery, vinegar, alcohol, and greasy fried foods. Bran should be added to the diet, and it is best to keep to three substantial meals a day with no snacking.

Note. Peppermint oil should not be used by persons diagnosed as lacking in hydrochloric acid (an acid secreted by the cells lining the stomach).

PAPAYA

Botanical Name: *Carica Papaya*
Common Names: Medicine Tree, Melon Tree

Papaya is a tropical, melon-like fruit produced in clusters by the *Carica papaya* tree. This handsome plant, which grows to a height of 20 feet, is crowned with tufts of leaves on long footstalks and is often referred to as the medicine tree or melon tree. In south China and other areas of the Far East where it was introduced less than a century ago, it is called Shu-kua, "tree melon," Wan-shou-kua, "longevity melon," and Fan-kua, "foreign melon."

Most of the papaya imported into the U.S. mainland comes from Hawaii, where the soil and climate is most suitable for the delicately flavored fruit.

Early Uses

Papaya is often mentioned in the writings of the early explorers. Columbus observed that the natives of the Caribbean could eat exceptionally heavy meals of fish and meat without apparent indigestion if the meal was followed by a dessert of papaya. Magellan regarded the fruit as a valuable component of the diet, and Marco Polo credited its use with saving the lives of his sailors when they were stricken with scurvy. Chester French told of the time he suffered agonizing stomach cramps which disappeared in an almost miraculous manner after he had eaten a papaya melon given to him by a Guatemalan native. In the sixteenth century, Spanish soldiers in Mexico serving with Cortez experienced relief from gastric discomfort by eating a slice of papaya.

Many of the early explorers also observed that the natives could tenderize tough meat by wrapping it in green papaya leaves overnight before cooking.

Modern Uses

The enzyme content of papaya is considerable, the most important being a broad-spectrum digestive enzyme called papain. Unlike other enzymes which perform only in an acid medium or solely in an alkaline medium, papain acts in all three—acid, alkaline, or neutral. It also performs on all three food groups—protein, fats, and carbohydrates. This ability gives it great importance as a digestive aid.

Papain enzyme tablets made from papaya fruit are available on the market. Along with their use for coping with indigestion, they have also proved successful in some instances for treating external hemorrhoids. One tablet is generally taken every three or four hours until the hemorrhoid conditioned has been remedied, which usually occurs within one week when it is effective. Papaya papain is also useful as an anthelmintic (destructive to intestinal worms).

Case Studies

One woman wrote: "Since using papaya fruit enzyme tablets, my tongue no longer has a white coating, and my digestion is ever so much better. I encouraged my brother to try the tablets, as he was often bothered by gas, belching, and heartburn as soon as he finished his meals. He is very grateful to the papaya tablets, for he is no longer troubled with indigestion."

A man found he could eat almost anything he wanted so long as he took his papaya enzyme tablets after each meal. He explained that he had been troubled with digestive disturbances symptomized by sour eructions, gas bloat, bad breath, and headaches, which he had previously controlled by adopting a very restrictive diet.

A physician reported the case of a 52-year-old woman who suffered terribly from painful external hemorrhoids. The patient was resistant to the idea of surgery, but as standard medical therapies produced no response the doctor instructed her to take one papain tablet every four hours. In 48 hours marked improvement was noted—the pain and swelling had subsided, and after three more days of the papain treatment the healing was complete. Surgery was not necessary.

CAROB

Botanical Name: *Ceratonia siliqua*
Common Names: St. John's Bread, Carob Pods, Carob Beans, Sugar Pods

This small evergreen tree is native to the coastal regions of the Mediterranean and produces seed pods which the Arabs call Kharoub (carob). The pods are also known as St. John's Bread, as they were eaten by John the Baptist during the time he spent in the wilderness.

Carob has a taste remarkably similar to that of chocolate, but far from creating problems such as chocolate can (e.g., allergies, poor teeth, nervousness), carob contributes to bodily health.

Reported Uses

During the Spanish Civil War (1936–1939) distressing outbreaks of diarrhea occurred which defied all efforts to contain it until a physician, Dr. Ramos, noticed that the condition was more prevalent among children of wealthy parents than those of the poor. He found that the poor children ate carob beans as a substitute for sweets. This led him to the discovery than carob, a highly nutritious food rich in vitamins and minerals, was curative for diarrhea.

Reports in medical journals during the 1950s showed that a powder made from carob had been accepted world-wide as a valuable, fast-acting antidiarrheal agent for infants, children, and adults. In the *Journal of Pediatrics* 1951, T. R. Ploweright described his experience in treating 40 cases of diarrhea among infants. All the infants were on antibiotics, and any of the fluid lost from diarrhea was replaced when necessary. One group of 20 infants was give carob powder added to their milk formulas, while the second group was not. In 48 hours, stools were formed in the first group, whereas it took 174 hours in the second group.

In another report, (*Canadian Medical Journal*, 1953), 230 cases of infants with diarrhea were treated with the addition of carob powder mixed in milk. All but three of the cases were cured.

A few years later, the *Bulletin of the Biological Sciences Foundation* (March-April, 1956) reported that in many European countries, carob powder "is almost routinely added to the formulas of infants as a measure for the prevention of loose stools." The *Bulletin* went on to say:

> Adult patients have been found to respond very favorably to carob, establishing it as a useful mode of treatment for ambulatory working persons. For example, in a recent series of 626 industrial workers with diarrhea, Devlin found that 1 to 5 doses (of a carob product) combatted 60% of 266 cases of infectious diarrhea, 95% of 220 cases of non-infectious diarrhea, and 99% of 140 cases of psychosomatic diarrhea. In only 15% of the infectious diarrhea was added specific therapy necessary.

Clues to the effectiveness of carob may be in the high amount of fibre it contains, which recent evidence demonstrates is helpful for digestive problems, including diarrhea. Carob is also a rich source of pectin, the substance which offers protection against loose stools.

PROPOLIS

Propolis is a sweet-smelling, resinous substance gathered by bees from the bark or leaf buds of trees, especially poplars. Its remedial value has been known for thousands of years as a treatment for numerous ailments. Today, interest in this natural healing substance has been revived, and its effectiveness is being scientifically verified in many parts of the world.

Constituents and Uses

According to Soviet medical research teams, propolis is classed as antibiotic and antiviral, with no side effects. It contains ample amounts of minerals and vitamins, particularly the B vitamins, along with organic and amino acids, pollen, essential oils, resin, wax, balsam, phytoncides, and other constituents.

Although many ailments respond favorably to propolis treatment, this wonderful substance is especially effective for stomach ulcers, skin problems, and infections of the mouth and throat.

Scientific Studies

In Austria, Dr. Franz K. Feiks at the Klosterneuburg Hospital tested propolis on patients with duodenal and gastric ulcers. One group was given standard medication, while the other group received drops of a 5% extract of propolis in water three times daily before meals. The group receiving the propolis were relieved of pain within three days, but only 10 of those on standard medication were relieved in the same amount of time. After 10 days, no wounds could be detected in 6 out of 10 patients using propolis.

Dr. Feiks also treated 15 outpatients with propolis. Hospitalization was required in only one case, whereas in another group of 17 patients who did not take propolis, 11 were subsequently hospitalized.

In other tests where patients were already hospitalized, Dr. Feiks employed propolis as a supplement to conventional medical treatment in 198 patients out of 294. Ninety percent of the propolis group were free of symptoms after two weeks.

Availability and Use of Propolis

Propolis is available in many forms (e.g., capsules, tinctures). In the condition of ulcers, one capsule is taken three times a day, about one-half hour before meals.

Note. Tests conducted at the Department of Dermatology Royal Infirmary, Edinburgh, Scotland, showed that one out of every 2,000 persons is allergic to propolis. Anyone who develops a rash after using the substance should stop the treatment. The rash reportedly disappears shortly after the propolis treatment has been discontinued.

CHINESE TRADITIONAL HERB FORMULAS

Following are some examples of herbal combinations used in Oriental medicine for treating certain gastrointestinal and bowel disorders. The herbs in these formulas are scientifically selected and carefully balanced in various proportions for maximum potency. The majority have been approved for use in medical facilities by the National Health Administration, Republic of China, and/or the Department of Pharmaceutical Affairs, Ministry of Health and Welfare, Japan. They are commercially available, and directions for their use are given on the labels of the bottles.

Pinellia Combination

Constituents: Pinellia, scute, coptis, ginseng, jujube, ginger, licorice.

Uses: Stagnancy below the sternum, borborygmus (rumbling noise caused by gas in the intestines), diarrhea with gastritis (inflammation of the stomach lining), gastroptosis (downward displacement of the stomach), and chronic dysentery; alternating diarrhea and constipation, or nausea, vomiting, and anorexia; gastrectasia; gastric ulcer; fermentive diarrhea.[4]

Pinellia and Ginseng Six Combination

Constituents: Pinellia, ginseng, scute, hoelen, oyster shell, ginger, atractylodes, coptis, licorice, citrus.

Stagnant heaviness in the stomach when hungry, and general malnutrition; gastroenteritis (inflammation of the stomach and intestines; cramps and diarrhea are characteristic symptoms); gastric ulcers; gastroptosis; stomachache; gastric spasms; abdominal pain; duodenal ulcers; and emaciated constitution.[5]

Cimfuga Combination

Constituents: Rhubarb, scute, tang-kuei, licorice root, bupleurum, cimicifuga.

Uses: Hemorrhoids, hemorrhoidal fissures, pain, and bleeding; the initial stages of anal prolapse, constipation; hard stools. The best formula in Chinese medication for hemorrhoids.[6]

Lithospermum Ointment

Constituents: Lithospermum, sesame oil, tang-kuei, flava, wax, lard.

Uses: Applied externally on hemorrhoids.[7]

Cardamon and Fennel Combination

Constituents: Cinnamon, cordyalis, fennel, oyster shell, lesser galanga, licorice, cardamon.

Uses: Gastritis, prolapsed and weak stomach, and gastric and duodenal ulcers.[8]

Apricot Seed and Linum Combination

Constituents: Linum, peony, chih-shih, magnolia, apricot seed, rhubarb.

Uses: A mild cathartic; for elderly people with general weakness or constipation during convalescence, habitual constipation (weakness), or hemorrhoids due to constipation.[9]

Pinellia and Gastrodia Combination

Constituents: Pinellia, atractylodes, citrus, hoelen, malt, gastrodia, ginger, shen-chu, astragalus, ginseng, alisma, phellodendron, dried ginger.

Uses: Weak gastrointestinal tract with paroxysmal headaches and vertigo, chills in the legs and feet, gastric atonia, gastroptosis, gastritis, neurosis, hypertension, suppuration.[10]

Pinellia and Magnolia Combination

Constituents: Pinellia, hoelen, magnolia bark, perilla, ginger.

Uses: To be taken for esophageal constriction and the sensation of foreign matter in the throat.[11]

Pinellia and Gardenia Combination

Constituents: Pinellia, scute, coptis, ginseng, jujube, ginger, licorice.

Uses: To be taken for esophogeal constriction and difficulty in swallowing.[12]

Coptis Combination

Constituents: Coptis, ginseng, pinellia, licorice, cinnamon, ginger, jujube.

Uses: To be taken for sensation of heavy pressure in the stomach, sour stomach, nausea, loss of appetite, and white coating on the tongue.[13]

Six Major Herb Combination

Constituents: Ginger, atractylodes, hoelen, pinellia, citrus, ginger, jujube, licorice.

Uses: Gastrointestinal weakness, food stagnancy with anorexia, nausea, stagnancy and fullness below the sternum, cold hands and feet due to anemia, gastroenteritis, gastritis, gastric weakness, dyspepsia, stomachache, vomiting, an emaciated constitution.[14]

SUMMARY

1. The effectiveness of herb remedies for treating certain gastrointestinal and bowel complaints has remained consistent over the ages.
2. Fenugreek is one of the finest of all herbal aids for cleansing the body of excessive mucus.
3. Peppermint tea is a timeless standby remedy for indigestion and resultant discomfort.
4. From earliest times papaya has been a valuable food source for promoting healthy digestion.
5. Along with an abundance of vitamins and minerals, papaya provides enzymes, the most important being papain.
6. Papain enzymes extracted from papaya are sold mainly as an aid for digestion; however, in some instances they have proved effective in conditions of external hemorrhoids.
7. Medical journals have reported that carob is a speedy antidiarrheal agent for infants, children, and adults.
8. A study in Australia showed that propolis has relieved many cases of gastric and duodenal ulcers.
9. There are a number of Chinese traditional herb formulas from which to choose for treating various gastrointestinal and bowel complaints.

ENDNOTES

1. *Grace*, Spring 1989.
2. *Grace*, Spring 1988.
3. *Grace*, Winter 1989.

4. Dr. Hong-Yen Hsu, *The Way to Good Health with Chinese Herbs* (Long Beach, CA: Oriental Healing Arts Institute, 1982).

5. Ibid.

6. Ibid.

7. Dr. Hong-Yen Hsu & Dr. Wm. G. Peacher, *Chinese Herb Medicine and Therapy* (Long Beach, CA: Oriental Healing Arts Institute, 1982).

8. Ibid.

9. Dr. Hong-Yen Hsu, *The Way to Good Health with Chinese Herbs* (Long Beach, CA: Oriental Healing Arts Institute, 1982.)

10. Ibid.

11. Dr. Hong-Yen Hsu, *How to Treat Yourself with Chinese Herbs* (Long Beach, CA: Oriental Healing Arts Institute, 1980).

12. Ibid.

13. Ibid.

14. Dr. Hong-Yen Hsu, *The Way to Good Health with Chinese Herbs* (Long Beach, CA: Oriental Healing Arts Institute, 1982).

C H A P T E R   8

HERBS FOR
THE BRAIN AND
CIRCULATORY SYSTEM

While some degree of memory difficulty occurs as we grow older, it is only when these difficulties become severe that the condition is termed senile dementia. But a great variation exists, as some people retain their faculties and abilities well into advanced years. Oliver Wendell Holmes at 79 wrote *Over the Teacups*; Goethe at 80 completed *Faust*; and Titian at 98 painted a masterpiece.

"Keep your mind going," doctors urge. "The brain as well as the body needs exercise."

Memory often deteriorates in senior citizens because of a growing constriction of interest. Elderly people may become bored and make no attempt to pay attention to what is going on around them or to accept and deal with new ideas and experiences. Finally the time arrives when, although the record of the events they have observed is still intact in the memory cells, the neural pathways of recall become "glossed over" and apparently lost.

Keep the Mind Young

One way to enhance the memory and thought processes is by activities which require attention and concentration. Reading books, writing letters, playing cards or chess, or working crossword puzzles are examples. The stimulation of new experiences, social contacts, a part-time job, or volunteer work can also help.

Two Main Types of Senile Dementia

According to medical experts, there are two main forms of senile dementia. One is a condition of intellectual impairment resulting from strokes or arterial disease. In some types of atherosclerotic dementia, the arteries of the brain become narrowed, restricting the blood flow and damaging brain tissues. The victim is often aware of memory lapses and becomes disoriented, which causes feelings of depression, anxiety, frustration, anger, and irritability.

The other is Alzheimer's disease, a tragic form of senility amply recorded by the German neurologist Alois Alzheimer. In this disease there is atrophy and shrinkage of the brain, but no atherosclerosis or blockage.

In Alzheimer's, changes most commonly occur in the proteins of the nerve cells in the part of the brain known as the cerebral cortex—the outer layer of the brain. The course of the disorder is very slow but relentless; symptoms include poor memory and disorientation. When the process continues year after year, mental deterioration becomes so drastic that victims are unable to care for themselves.

Alzheimer's Cases Increasing

Dr. Denis Evans of Brigham and Women's Hospital conducted a study of 3,623 people living in Boston. He reports that 47.2% of people over the age of 85 may have Alzheimer's in contrast with previous estimates of 20%. "People over 85 are the fastest growing age group in the U.S.," he points out. All in all, he found that 1 in 10 people over 65 appear to have the disease.

What this means, according to Dr. Teresa Radebaugh of the National Institute on Aging in Bethesda, Maryland, is that current estimates of Alzheimer's cases should be upscaled to nearly 4 million people from the previous 2.5 million. She explains that the study, which appeared in the *Journal of the American Medical Association*, is one of the first to look at Alzheimer's in the general population. Estimates taken earlier were not as accurate because they were based on patients in institutions. Fourteen million people are predicted to have the disease by the year 2040, according to the Alzheimer's Disease and Related Disorders Association.[1]

The Alzheimer-Aluminum Connection

For some years, aluminum has been implicated as a possible cause of Alzheimer's disease. A Canadian investigator working on post-mortems found higher than normal levels of this metal in the brains of patients who had died of the disease. Through imperfect elimination, aluminum salts are found deposited in the brain and other tissues, resulting in the mental deterioration of the sufferers.

According to a study published in *The Lancet*[2], a British medical journal, people living in areas with high concentrations of aluminum in drinking water had a greater risk of contracting Alzheimer's. The Medical Research Council said the risk of getting the disease increased up to 50% with higher levels of the metal in drinking water.

Experiments with lab animals treated with aluminum demonstrated a response somewhat akin to dementia, along with changes in behavior similar to those observed in humans with Alzheimer's.

The Increasing Use of Aluminum

In former times people never heard of Alzheimer's disease. In those days aluminum salts were rarely used, except as a pickling agent for vegetables. Today, aluminum is in cookware, tap water, and aerosols. It is added to numerous foods and medicinals. It appears in processed cheeses as an emulsifying agent. One slice can contain two-and-a-half times the average person's daily intake. Examples of other sources are cake mixtures, baking powders, and antacids (alkali salts for the relief of indigestion, acidity, etc.).

There are aluminum cans—remember when soft drinks and beer were sold only in bottles? There is also aluminum foil, a common household item used to wrap food. Commercial frozen foods are packaged in aluminum as well.

Since it is impossible to control all of these sources, it is necessary to make every attempt to eliminate those over which we do have control. For example: We should replace aluminum cookware with stainless steel, Pyrex®, or enamel; use bottled spring water instead of tap water; read all labels on packaged or canned food products and medicinals; and purchase beverages in bottles whenever possible.

It may take years before aluminum build-up reaches the degree in the body where symptoms of Alzheimer's are in evidence. Regrettably, that point has already been reached for many people, and the disease is steadily on the rise.

Although science has not yet proven conclusively that exposure to aluminum causes Alzheimer's or why some people more that others are prone to the metal's toxic effects, there is no need to take chances. Exposure to aluminum should be avoided as much as possible.

What Else Can Be Done?

Dr. Bartram writes:

> Once aluminum has been layed down in placque form in the brain it is difficult to understand how it can be resolved. Such elderly patients are most likely to suffer from deficiency of calcium; this puts them at risk in laying down more aluminum. While the first consideration is to avoid the source of contamination, the new technique of chelation appears to be indicated. To facilitate elimination of aluminum salts, a 48 hour fluid-only fast each month for six months should assist. Improvement has been reported by large doses of vitamin B Complex.[3]

Dr. Bartram also mentions the use of herbs as being important.

In addition a good basic diet with supplemental vitamins, minerals, and amino acids helps to control and prevent senile dementia, according to nutritionally oriented physicians. Drinking enough water (eight glasses a day) is also advised, as inadequate amounts of fluids can result in dehydration. Exercise is important too, as increased blood flow brings oxygen to the brain.

Physicians point out that diagnosis of senile dementia should be done as soon as possible, as treatment is more likely to be effective at that time.

HERBS FOR MENTAL AND CIRCULATORY HEALTH

The herbs discussed in this chapter have reportedly proved helpful in coping with conditions relating to aging and circulation.

GINKGO TREE

Botanical Name: *Ginkgo biloba*
Common Name: Ginkgo

The name Ginkgo is derived from the Japanese pronunciation of two characters, Yin-Kuo.

The ginkgo is one of the oldest living species of trees and can be traced back more than 200 million years. It is a tall tree, up to 100 feet high, with a trunk 18 to 20 feet or more in girth. Its fan-shaped, bilobed leaves are light green in color when young, darker toward mid-summer, and golden in autumn. The orange-yellow seeds have a fleshy outer covering resembling a small plum.

Ginkgo is commonly planted in China, Manchuria, and Japan, especially in the grounds of Buddhist temples, where magnificent specimens were reported to be over 1,000 years old. It is also cultivated in Europe and the United States, where it has become familiar to tree lovers everywhere, not only for its great beauty but also because of its remarkable immunity to insects, disease, and pollution.

Ginkgo has been employed in Oriental medicine for thousands of years.

Modern Remedial Uses

An extract of ginkgo leaves has demonstrated positive effects on different parts of the circulatory and nervous systems. It increased blood flow to the brain, nerve signal transmission, cellular energy production, free radical scavenging activity, and may also offer protection against stroke.

In Europe the extract has been recommended as a supplement to resist the effects of premature aging and for individuals with symptoms of aging such as short-term memory loss, senility, inattentiveness, stress-related depression, and tinnitus (ringing in the ears). Its use appears to improve memory, immunity, circulatory ills, and overall mental energy, performance, awareness, and attentiveness.

Tens of millions of bottles of ginkgo extract have been sold in Europe over the past years.

Cerebral Vascular Insufficiency. Numerous scientific studies in Europe have been undertaken with the use of ginkgo for cerebral vascular insufficiency (decreased blood flow to the brain), a condition often seen in people as a result of atherosclerosis.

In one representative study,[4] 112 geriatric patients suffering from chronic cerebral insufficiency received 40 milligrams of ginkgo extract three times a day for one year. The ages of the patients ranged for 55 to 94. Results showed that symptoms of short-term memory loss, headaches, vertigo, (dizziness), depression, inability to concentrate, and tinnitus were alleviated.

In a French study,[5] 103 tinnitus out-patients were treated during a 13-month period by 10 specialists using a double-blind study method of ginkgo extract versus a placebo. All the tinnitus patient using the extract improved.

In *Nutrition News*,[6] we find the following:

An overview of literature in *Medical News* states: "Ginkgo is particularly effective in delaying the mental deterioration of patients in just beginning to experience cognitive defects. Gingko helps these patients halt their deterioration and to avoid institutionalization." In a study documented by dynamic brain mapping (using EEGs), Fungfeld and Stalleiken found that mental alertness increased dramatically with ginkgo therapy.

Intermittent Claudication. Intermittent claudication also responds to ginkgo extract. This is a condition resulting from narrowed arteries in the leg, symptomized by pain or weakness in the leg or foot when walking. A six-month double-blind study[7] of 79 patients troubled with peripheral arterial insufficiency of the leg was conducted. Thirty-five patients were treated with a placebo and 44 with coated tablets containing 40 milligrams ginkgo biloba extract: Rökan®.

The two groups were comparable in weight, age, height, risk factors, and proportions of male to female patients. The average age was 60.9. There was a dramatic increase in pain-free walking distance and maximum distance walked in the group taking the ginkgo extract compared to the placebo group.

Anti– Free-Radical Action of Ginkgo. A free radical is a fragment of a molecule that has been torn away from its source and tends to join the body's normal molecules, where it can seriously damage or even cause a chain reaction of molecular destruction. Cells die, enzymes fail to function, energy is reduced, and the body's ability to renew itself and resist and recover from illness is diminished.

The destructive reaction caused by free radicals can be almost completely suppressed by antioxidants. Ginkgo possesses antioxidant action and has demonstrated a powerful free radical scavenging effect.[8]

Cholesterol. *Nutrition News*[9] reports: "In one Chinese study, 88 patients with an average total cholesterol of 236, lowered their count to an average of 197 in one to three months daily ginkgo extract."

Extended Power of Ginkgo. Conditions relating to circulatory problems and aging are not the only areas in which ginkgo has proved effective. Many healthy users of the herbal extract experienced marked enhancement of memory and mental alertness.

In one clinical study the reaction time in healthy young women taking a memory test improved remarkably after receiving ginkgo biloba extract.[10]

Other healthy users of the extract have also reported beneficial results. For example, during his research one man found the herb especially effective for long-term studying when mental clarity begins to diminish with time. He recommends that students take ginkgo "one-half hour to an hour ahead of the mental workout." He explains, "It helps you to be more focused on what you're studying."[11]

How Ginkgo Is Used

Many fine ginkgo biloba products in various forms such as extracts, powders, capsules, and tablets are available from health food stores and herb firms.

The standard dose of 40 milligrams in solid extract form (24%) is taken three times a day, making a total of 120 milligrams daily. However, it can range to 240 milligrams three times daily. It is necessary to take the doses throughout the day, as ginkgo passes very quickly through the body.

Although quite rare, mild adverse reactions of intestinal upset and headache have been reported.

Ginkgo is also available on the market in combination with other herbs known to improve mental performance such as ginseng and gotu-kola.

HAWTHORN

Botanical Name: *Crataegus oxycantha*
Common Names: May Blossom, May Bush, English Hawthorn, Haw

The white or pink-flowered hawthorn tree is native to Europe, Africa, and Asia but has been naturalized in many other parts of the world. Its brilliant red berries with yellow pulp hang in clusters from thorny branches and remain on the tree after the leaves drop off in autumn.

In country villages people claimed they could predict a mild or cold winter depending on the crop of berries the hawthorn produced. A heavy crop denoted cold winter months ahead; the abundance of berries would serve as food for the birds who had not flown south to a warmer climate. Few berries meant a mild winter.

In France the hawthorn was formerly regarded as sacred, for it was believed to be the tree from which Christ's crown of thorns was made. In Greece and Rome it symbolized marriage and fertility. At weddings the vases at the nuptial altar were filled with fragrant hawthorn flowers, and brides were adorned with the blossoms.

Early Remedial Discovery of Hawthorn

John Wesley, in the eighteenth century, not only devoted his time to the spiritual needs of his followers but also to their health problems, and to this end he used the herbs of the fields. It is due to his keen observations that medical herbalists learned much of the value of hawthorn as a heart tonic.

Wesley reportedly noticed that when many of the horses he had ridden so hard became winded and exhausted, they would immediately eat hawthorn berries when turned loose into country paddocks. In a short time they recovered and were able to take him to a further parish for more sermons. Even a horse that had been pronounced "broken winded" would make an excellent recovery after eating hawthorn berries. Wesley then began using the berries with excellent results as a heart tonic and heart remedy for humans.

Modern Uses

Hawthorn is classed a cardiac, tonic, antispasmodic, and sedative.

In herbal medicine, preparations of hawthorn berry cover a wide range of heart conditions. They are used in cases of weak heart muscle, inflammation of the heart, irregular heartbeat, nervous heart problems, high blood pressure, and atherosclerosis.

A Medical Opinion of Hawthorn

Dr. Eric Powell, who has used hawthorn in his medical practice for many years, has this to say about its value:[12]

> The Hawthorn berry in any medicinal form is probably the finest general heart tonic ever discovered. It is absolutely harmless and can only do good. Will never be contra-indicated in any type of heart affected, although in some instances other remedies may be called for. An ideal natural remedy for failing compensation, irregular heart, circulatory trouble, congestion of the medulla oblongata, high blood pressure, the insomnia of heart sufferers, anxiety, and irritability. Valuable in valvular weakness and lack of tone in the muscle of the heart. Excellent for heart collapse due to typhoid and general debility. Helps to clear foreign deposits from arterial walls. A remedy for cardiac dropsy. The pulse may be irregular, feeble, or accelerated. Fatty degeneration has responded to crataegus (hawthorn), and it may be said that the remedy sustains the heart in all debilitating and infectious diseases.

An Impressive Case Study

Frank Roberts, F.N.I.M.H., writes:[13] "I would mention the case of a patient of mine whose heart's action was so strident and turbulent that I could hear all I needed to while he was sitting five or six feet away from me; within 14 days fluid extract of hawthorn had so quieted his heart that I had to use a stethoscope to hear what was going on; the tremendous pulsing of his collar, tie and shirt front had completely subsided."

Methods of Using Hawthorn

Eight to 15 drops of the extract of hawthorn berries are taken in a little warm or cold water three times daily before meals. For young children, five drops are sufficient according to medical herbalists.

If the homeopathic form is used instead, the tiny pills may be taken in the third or thirtieth potency. However, Dr. Powell states:[14] "Experience leads us to prefer the 30th potency, although excellent results follow the 3x. For the 30th potency take 5 pills on rising and 5 on retiring daily."

SOYBEAN LECITHIN

Lecithin is an incredible food with an astonishing range of important functions in the maintenance of good health and well-being. However, in this chapter we will limit our attention to its functions as a brain tonic and emulsifier.

Lecithin: Food for the Brain

In the brain, lecithin choline is transformed into acetylcholine, a chemical component which directly influences certain brain messages or neurotransmitters. This discovery was made in 1975 by scientists at the Massachusetts Institute of Technology. The most remarkable aspect of the discovery was that the brain has the ability to take up choline directly from the circulating blood. It has long been thought that something called the "brain barrier" protects the brain from direct influences. Previously it was believed that only a few substances, mainly narcotics and alcohol, could get through the barrier. But lecithin choline can do so, too, which means that with the use of lecithin as a dietary supplement, there can be an immediate effect of the production of chemical signals in the brain. This has shown a definite and beneficial effect on memory, thinking ability, and muscle control.

The Emulsifying Power of Lecithin

Lecithin helps prevent cholesterol and other fats from accumulating in the walls of the arteries and also helps to dissolve any deposits that may already be there. A build-up of these dangerous fatty deposits can plug the blood vessels and could result in atherosclerosis and heart attacks. The greater amount of saturated fat in the blood, the more likely it is to clot, which may lead to phlebitis, stroke, coronary thrombosis, or a pulmonary embolism.

Dr. Richard Carleton, chairman of the National Cholesterol Education Program, says the link between blood cholesterol and heart disease is "enormous and compelling." He cites the following statistics: Over 6 million Americans have heart disease symptoms. Each year, about 1.25 million suffer heart attacks; 500,000 die. About 55% of U.S. adults have cholesterol levels that are borderline or higher (200 milligrams or more); 25% are in the high range (above 240).[15]

In her book *Let's Get Well,*[16] Adele Davis reports:

> All atherosclerosis is characterized by an increase of blood cholesterol and a *decrease in lecithin*. As early as 1935 it was shown that experimental heart disease, produced by feeding cholesterol, could be prevented merely by giving a small amount of lecithin; and atherosclerosis has since been repeatedly produced in various species either by decreasing the blood lecithin or increasing cholesterol. If enough lecithin is given, the disease does not occur regardless of how much cholesterol is fed. Even when atherosclerosis is far advanced, health is restored after lecithin is supplied in the diet.

Davis also reports that within three months, the blood cholesterol level of patients who had suffered heart attacks dropped markedly after they took 4 to 6 tablespoons of lecithin daily. In one case the level was reduced from 1,012 to 186 milligrams. The patients were relieved of pain and other symptoms and felt much better. Once the cholesterol levels became normal, the amount of lecithin was reduced to 1 to 2 tablespoons a day. Davis adds: "Supplements of lecithin have also caused angina pains to disappear and have been especially beneficial to elderly patients who have suffered stroke, or have cerebral atherosclerosis."

Case Studies

Dr. Lester Morrison reported a clinical study[17] of 15 men and women between the ages of 38 and 80 who had been unsuccessfully treated for high blood cholesterol levels for up to 10 years. After taking 2 tablespoons of lecithin three times daily with meals for three months, 12 of the 15 patients experienced an average reduction of 156 milligrams of serum cholesterol. Two of the patients had a history of angina pains, but after using lecithin, the angina symptoms vanished. No other treatment was given to reduce the cholesterol levels.

The amount of lecithin taken by the patients was a total of 6 tablespoons daily, but follow-up work indicated that a maintenance dose of 1 to 2 tablespoons per day was effective in sustaining normal cholesterol levels. Dr. Morrison says that lecithin "is an exceptionally valuable bulwark against 'hardening of the arteries' and all the complications of heart, brain and kidney that follow."

BLACKSTRAP MOLASSES

Blackstrap molasses is the nutritive dark, thick, syrup that is left when refined sugar is made from sugar cane. This natural food is rich in mineral salts and most of the vitamin B complex.

Herbalists and naturopaths value the daily use of blackstrap molasses for clearing up or preventing many disorders, including heart and circulatory problems. For example, it reportedly strengthens the heart muscles, reduces high blood pressure, remedies varicose veins, and keeps fat on the move, preventing it from adhering to the walls of the arteries. Some cases have been reported where strokes have yielded to molasses therapy.

Method of Using Molasses

Blackstrap molasses may be taken before, during, or after meals, or whenever most convenient. One teaspoonful is dissolved in half a cup of hot water. Then cold water is added to make two-thirds of a cup, drank warm.

The beverage should not be gulped down, but sipped slowly. Persons with delicate stomachs who find a teaspoonful too much are advised to use smaller doses, taken more often during the day.

Case Studies

Mrs. W. W. writes: "I would like to say that after 18 years of suffering from poor circulation and varicose veins, and ulcers that got worse all the time, I had the vein in my left leg stripped. However, after a month or so, it began to swell again.

"Then I read a book about molasses and started taking one teaspoonful a day in a little water. That was 19 years ago. I have never had any vein trouble since, although I worked in a hospital and was on my feet all the time.

"Apparently molasses strengthens the walls of the veins and, according to the writer of the book, acts against cancer also. Where the cane sugar is harvested in the West Indies it is chewed by the laborers and cancer is almost unknown. One thing I do know, molasses has done me so much good in so many ways. I would not give up taking it."

Author Cyril Scott of England reports:[19] "Mr. X, an elderly man, suffered two strokes and was completely paralyzed down one side of his body. He then tried molasses therapy—with the gratifying results the he *recovered the use of all his limbs,* and became completely fit, much to the astonishment of his doctor and friends. Nor is this by any means an isolated case, and if I have selected it out of many others, it is because it happens to be a particularly bad one.

"The question of paralytic strokes gives one much food for reflection, and I think it is not too far to say that if people would make molasses part of their daily diet there might be fewer cases of this dreadful affliction."

Another of the cases Scott reports[20] concerns that of cardiac thrombosis (blood clot). He writes: "The sufferer was a railway worker who had been obliged to give up his job for life owing to his condition. He was induced to try the molasses and was so pleased with the results that he was able to go back to work—a fit man. The potassium and other mineral salts in the aliment had dispersed the clot."

Note. Diabetics should not use molasses.

GINSENG

Botanical Name: *Panax schinseng*
Common Names: Man-Plant, Root of Life, Long Life Root, Wonder Root, Flower of Life

Asiatic ginseng is a small perennial herb with five palmate leaves, minute yellowish-green flowers in an umbrellate form, and red berry-like fruits. It resembles the North American ginseng, *Panax quinquefolium*, which is native to the eastern half of the U.S. and southern Canada. Another variety is know as Tienchi ginseng, *Panax notoginseng*. All these plants have essentially the same properties.

The term *Panax* is taken from the Greek *panakeia*, the word source for *panacea*, in reference to the alleged cure-all powers of the herb.

Cultivation of Ginseng

Asiatic ginseng grows wild in shaded mountainous regions of the Far East but is now rare, as it has been hunted almost out of existence. Consequently, the world market depends on the cultivated plants, and the Koreans reportedly were the first to perfect the technique of growing the herb commercially. There the government strictly regulates the cultivation and production of ginseng, and Koreans give very careful attention to the crops. After harvest the roots are cleaned, steamed to make red ginseng, and dried naturally for white ginseng. The red ginseng is of exceptionally high quality and carries a government seal with a registered trademark.

A very fine quality of American ginseng is grown in Wisconsin.

Man-Plant

The term *ginseng* in Chinese characters means "man-like," and often the shape of the root somewhat resembles the human figure. Numerous legends relating to this peculiarity of shape can be found in ancient Oriental writings. One quaint legend from early Chinese work declares: "The plant, after growing for three centuries, is inspired through the star-light by the Spirits of the hills and rivers, then bursts into the shape and form of a man. In the course of time the new creature can leave the earth and dwell among the stars; but the most wonderful part about him is his white blood, which is a sovereign cure for all diseases and a safe-guard against mortality."

Early Uses of Ginseng

Literature on the use of ginseng in China dates from the earliest times. Of these works the oldest is the *Pen Ts'ao Ching*, in which Emperor Shen-Nung described various medicaments with instructions for their use. Among the herbs covered in the pharmacopeia, ginseng is rated the highest and most potent. Shen-Nung claimed the root was a valuable tonic which produced a beneficial effect on the eyes and brain, and that if taken for some time it would invigorate the body and prolong life.

Subsequent editions of Shen-Nung's pharmacopeia were ordered during the Han dynasty (A.D. 206–220), again in the Tang dynasty (A.D. 618–907), and the latest, still in print, in 1596 under the Ming dynasty.

In the sixteenth century, Li Shih Chen, physician and pharmacologist, spent 30 years compiling a massive work called the *Pen Ts'ao Kang Mu*, which included remedies from previous eras together with his own discoveries. In this book, Jen-shen (ginseng) is listed as an excellent physical restorative.

The pharmacopeia of Li Shih Chen is till considered highly important in the Far East. In 1956, the People's Republic of China issued a postage stamp in Li Shih Chen's honor.

Early information on the value of ginseng can also be found widely scattered in old almanacs, journals of travelers, botanists' field notes, and records of missionaries, all claiming that the use of ginseng increases vitality, invigorates the system, restores health, and prolongs life.

Modern Usage

Soviet scientists have been conducting research on Chinese and Korean ginseng since 1949, and seven volumes have been published by a special Ginseng Committee. Since then, the Committee has held 23 sessions in which Soviet and foreign scientists participated.

To summarize briefly, the results of these intensive studies have established that ginseng

- Improves the work of the brain cells
- Has a mild stabilizing effect on the blood pressure whether high or low
- Relieves atherosclerosis
- Improves memory
- Strengthens the body's defense system
- Increases physical endurance and stamina
- Has a safe, natural stimulating effect especially in tired and weak patients
- Improves vision and hearing acuity
- Reduces blood cholesterol
- Stimulates the functions of the endocrine glands
- Produces a good effect in a number of disorders of the central nervous system including neurasthenia and various neuroses

- Enhances the effectiveness of other treatments in cases of diabetes, diseases of the liver, impotence and several other ailments

Although the list is a long one, Professor Israel Brekhman states that ginseng is not a cure-all. He explains that "ginseng being a good tonic, a roborant, increases resistance of the organism and helps it to overcome many diseases of various origins."

Ginseng meets all the standards of an adaptogen and also possesses antiradical and antioxidant action.

Other Reported Uses of Ginseng

Professor Finn Sandberg conducted one of the first documented ginseng tests on volunteers in western Europe. To test its effect on the powers of concentration, he gave ginseng daily to some of the students for over a period of 33 days. This was done as a double blind test so that none of the students knew which of them had taken a placebo and which had taken ginseng. Those using the ginseng made significantly fewer mistakes in a complicated letter-canceling test and a spiral-maze test. Professor Sandberg concluded that ginseng demonstrated a "significant positive effect on psychomotor activity and simultaneous capacity."[21]

Nutrition News reports:

> In 1972 a study on clinical observations was published by the Medical Institute Centre Hospitalier, Argenteuil, France. A combination of ginseng, vitamins and trace minerals was given to 145 cases. "In cases of aged patients who present troubles of aging with diminished intellectual output, loss of memory and slow thinking, the therapeutic effect of ginseng was seen after one week of treatment and a considerable improvement noted during treatment for two months."

Tienchi ginseng reportedly produces a beneficial effect on the circulatory system, especially for problems of the veins and arteries.

Tests at the Beijing Institute of Physical Culture demonstrated that tienchi strengthens the constitution and improves the functions of the cardiovascular system. Trials with operation personnel at the high altitude of the Tibetan plateau showed that those who took tienchi ginseng did not experience irregular heart beat whereas the others had irregular changes in their electrocardiograms.

Six hundred and eighty hospital patients suffering from coronary disease and angina pectoris were given a clinical preparation of processed tienchi ginseng for 2 months. The beneficial rate effect was 60–95 percent and electrocardiogram improvements were 40–50 percent. Tienchi was found to reduce the number of attacks of angina patients and quickly eliminate or alleviate the symptoms. Patients who depended on nitroglycerine tablets were able to reduce the dosage.[23]

Methods of Using Ginseng

Ginseng can be purchased in many forms: the dried root, teabags, capsules, tinctures, fluid extracts, bulk powder, tiny envelopes of powdered ginseng, or as a blend or compound with other natural ingredients. One of the many examples is the product called Song Bao Su, a compound of ginseng extract with royal jelly.

Tienchi ginseng is also available on the market but is used only in processed form, never raw. One such Chinese product is called Tian Qi Pian, which consists of processed slices of tienchi root. The contents of one box of Tian Qi Pian is about 2-2/3 ounces. The Chinese prepare it for use by cooking half of the contents with chicken soup and simmering it slowly for two or three hours.

GARLIC

Botanical Name: *Allium sativa*
Common Name: Poor Man's Treacle

Garlic is rich in organic selenium and germanium along with sulphur compounds which are uniquely beneficial to cardiovascular physiology and the body's defense system.

Professor Hans Reuter[24] of Cologne, West Germany, has found that garlic helps clear fat accumulating in the blood vessels of people who like to eat rich food, thereby reducing the risk of heart attacks and strokes. A test demonstrated that volunteers fed butter containing 50 grams of garlic oil in gelatine capsules experienced a considerably lower level of cholesterol than a group fed butter without garlic. In a second test, patients ate 3 grams of raw garlic every day for four weeks, after which time their cholesterol level had dropped significantly.

According to Professor Reuter, not only does garlic drive out unwanted fats, but further tests showed that in some cases it is more effective than penicillin and other antibiotics. He also points out that in countries such as Japan, Russia, Korea, Greece, and India where garlic is commonly consumed, there are fewer cases of atherosclerosis, stroke, and other manifestations of hardening of the arteries.

Dr. Martyn Bailey of George Washington University in Washington, D.C., has shown that an anticlotting agent in garlic helps prevent the formation of potentially dangerous blood clots.

Methods of Using Garlic

Garlic is best taken in raw form, crushed or chopped—usually one clove per day mixed with food (e.g., salad, soup), although some people use more. However, chemist Eric Block of the State University of New York at Albany explains:[25] "Garlic does contain irritants, so people with hernias or stomach disorders—the elderly, for instance—should avoid eating lots of it. Overall, though, there isn't much evidence that normal amounts of garlic are bad for you."

Other forms of garlic, including tablets or capsules, should be used according to directions on the labels.

Kyolic® Garlic Extract

An editorial in the *Journal of the Indiana State Medical Association* (1982) states: "A Japanese developed garlic extract called Kyolic® is recommended for preventing heart disease and atherosclerosis, for maintaining cholesterol levels in normal range and for improving the body's immune system. The extract does not cause any unpleasant side effects. Added benefits are the lowering of blood sugar in diabetes and the raising of blood sugar in hypoglycemia."

Liquid Kyolic® garlic is cold-aged processed whole clove garlic devoid of the irritants of raw garlic. It is also available in combination with other nutritious substances. One example is *Formula 104*, which consists of Kyolic® garlic extract powder with the multiple benefits of lecithin. Another, Kyolic® *Formula 106*, combines garlic extract with vitamin E, hawthorn berry, and cayenne. Vitamin E is an important antioxidant/anti-free radical which bolsters the body's defense system; hawthorn berry is highly beneficial to cardiovascular health; traditionally, cayenne has been used for promoting peripheral circulation.

Directions for using these products are given on the labels.

OTHER HERBS FOR ENHANCING BRAIN AND CIRCULATORY FUNCTIONS

There are many other herbs which have demonstrated beneficial effects for the conditions cited in this chapter, among which are the following:

Eleuthero (Eleutherococcus senticosis). Commonly called Siberian ginseng. Has the same remarkable benefits as Panax ginseng but stronger action as a tonic and adaptogen and with a wider range of therapeutic activity. (See chapters 1 and 10.)

Suma® (Pfaffia paniculata). Enhances energy and vitality and shows great promise as a healing agent in chronic disorders believed to result from a lowered immune response.

Royal Jelly (Substance produced by young worker honey bees). Acts as a tonic. Improves memory and helps prevent premature senility. Has enabled nervous patients to respond with a more stable nervous system and a higher degree of stamina for mental and physical work.

Bee Pollen (A fine powder which forms inside the blossoms of flowering plants). Has health-building and regenerative properties. Builds strength and energy, fortifies the body against illnesses.

Minor Bupleurum Combination. Slows the aging process caused by free radicals.

Honey. Considered the best food for the heart. Used for heart and muscle weakness. In some countries it is said to be effective for dispersing fluid from around the heart. Also controls cramps in the legs or feet.

Song Bao Su. This Chinese product consists of Panax ginseng and royal jelly. Taken regularly it acts as a general health tonic which assists memory and circulation. Increases bodily resistance to some of the major effects of aging.

Yunnan Paiyao. Yunnan is the name of the border province in Southwest China; Pai means white; Yao means herb or medicine. According to Chinese herbalists, one particular function of Yunnan Paiyao which as yet is not widely known, is that of an effective remedy for strokes.

Gotu Kola (Centella asiatica). Used in India to treat fading memory, brain fatigue, depression, exhaustion, stuttering, and other chronic nervous disorders. It is also used for rheumatism, fevers, skin ailments, and many other conditions. (At one time it was believed to be a remedy for leprosy but is not considered a specific but only useful in ameliorating the symptoms and improving general health.)

SUMMARY

1. There are two main forms of senile dementia; one is intellectual impairment resulting from strokes or arterial disease, and the other is Alzheimer's.

2. For some years, overexposure to aluminum in food, water, etc. has been implicated as a possible cause of Alzheimer's disease.

3. Diagnosis of senile dementia should be conducted as soon as possible, as treatment is more likely to succeed at that time.

4. Ginkgo biloba extract has demonstrated positive effects on different parts of the circulatory and nervous systems and provides nutritional support to individuals with symptoms of aging. Intermittent claudication also responds to ginkgo extract.

5. The possibility of treating Alzheimer's disease with extract of ginkgo has been suggested by research conducted in France.

6. Hawthorn berry extract is valued as an effective heart tonic as well as a remedy for a wide range of heart problems.

7. Soybean lecithin is a key nutrient for the brain and also provides highly beneficial polyunsaturated fatty acids.

8. Blackstrap molasses reportedly prevents or remedies many disorders including heart and circulatory ills.

9. A beverage of blackstrap molasses should be sipped slowly.

10. Diabetics should not use molasses.

11. Panax ginseng is a prominent tonic which meets the standards of an adaptogen, affecting the total organism in a positive therapeutic way.

12. Studies have shown that tienchi ginseng has a beneficial effect on the circulatory system, especially for problems of the arteries and veins.

13. Tienchi ginseng should be used only in processed form, never raw.

14. Research shows that garlic possesses certain constituents which are uniquely therapeutic to cardiovascular physiology and the body's immune system.

15. Nature offers a treasury of additional herbs for the brain and circulatory system.

ENDNOTES

1. Tim Friend, *USA Today*, Nov. 10–12, 1989.
2. January 1989.
3. *Grace*, Summer 1986.

4. G. Vorberg, *Clinical Trials Journal*, 1985.

5. *La Presse Médical*, 1986.

6. Vol. XII, No. 10, 1989.

7. U. Bauer, *Arzneim Forsch.*, 1984.

8. S. S. Chatterjee & B. Gabard, *Naunyn-Schmiederberg's Arch. Pharmacol*, Vol. 320, 1982, p. R52.

9. Vol. XII, No. 10, 1989.

10. I. Hendmarch & Subbanz, *Int. J. Clin. Pharmacol*, 1984.

11. *Whole Foods*, December 1988.

12. *Building a Healthy Heart* (Rustington, Sussex, England: Health Science Press).

13. *Health from Herbs*, Jan.-Feb. 1968, Vol. 3, No. 15.

14. *Building a Healthy Heart* (Rustington, Sussex, England: Health Science Press).

15. Dan Sperling, *USA Today*, Feb. 28, 1990.

16. New York: Harcourt, Brace & World.

17. *The Low Fat Way to Health and Longer Life* (Englewood Cliffs, N.J.: Prentice-Hall).

18. *Grace*, Spring 1985.

19. *Crude Black Molasses* (Wellingborough, England: Athene Publishing Co., Ltd.).

20. Ibid.

21. *Health Digest*, Vol. 1, No. 7, 1979.

22. Vol. III, No. 12. 1980.

23. *Bestways*, February 1980.

24. *The Doctor*, November 1978.

25. *Hippocrates*, Jan.-Feb. 1985.

CHAPTER 9

NATURAL REMEDIES FOR SKIN PROBLEMS

Mrs. E. M. of Bermuda writes: "I am going to tell you a true story that happened to me a few weeks ago. A young friend from Australia was staying with us. We went for a swim off the end of our garden (we live on the sea edge), and whilst swimming I was stung badly by a Portuguese man-of-war jellyfish. I warned Campbell, but he was doing the Australian crawl and went into the same jellyfish. The tentacles were wrapped around his body and legs, and he was badly stung. We got out of the water, and I felt here was a chance to try an experiment. We had both been stung by the same jellyfish, so I ran up to the house and got a lemon and made him squeeze the juice on all the stings and let it dry. I did not use anything.

"That night it was painful, and I must have scratched the irritation for hours on end. The next morning my stings were red and angry and uncomfortable. Campbell had little pinpricks where the stings had been, but *no* irritation whatsoever and *no* pains.

"Two days after all this I fell into a bed of stinging nettles, and my knees were covered with the stings. Again my thoughts turned to lemon and I rushed inside, poured the juice on, and within *two seconds* all the sting had gone and never returned. I feel this is a tip worth knowing, especially for children.

"So now I am waiting for someone to get stung by a bee or hornet and let me see if the lemon works. I am sure it will."

The Miraculous Lemon

Of all foods which have been used as medicinal aids, the lemon is the most commonly known. Many illnesses including colds, sore throat, sinus trouble, biliousness, and headaches have effectively responded to its use. Even the custom of using a slice of lemon when eating a fish dinner was originally intended for remedial purposes rather than for flavoring. It was believed that if a fish bone was unknowingly swallowed during a meal, the juice of the lemon would dissolve it.

A Time-Tested Remedy

As time-tested home remedies for problems involving the skin, lemons are used as follows.

Chilblains. (1) Frequent applications of lemon juice mixed with glycerine are considered excellent for treating chilblains. (2) Half a lemon dipped in salt and rubbed on an unbroken chilblain reportedly gives almost immediate relief.

Insect Stings and Bites. Local applications of lemon juice are used to allay the irritation caused by bee or hornet stings and the bite of gnats and similar insects. Also effectively treats nettle inflammation.

Warts. The inner rind of a lemon is steeped in vinegar for 24 hours and then bandaged to the wart. The lemon rind must not remain on the wart more than three hours. It is applied fresh every day until results are achieved.

Corns and Calluses. The feet are soaked in hot water just before bedtime. After they are thoroughly dried, a small piece of lemon peeling with the pulp intact is bound over the corn or callus and bandaged. This is left on overnight and removed in the morning. The same procedure is repeated for four or five days, after which time the skin growth may be removed.

Black Heads. Lemon juice is applied to the area and allowed to dry.

Felon. The end of a lemon is cut off, and the finger which has the felon is inserted into the lemon and bound on. In the morning the matter will be drawn out almost to the surface, where it can be removed. When used in time, it reportedly scatters the felon.

Skin Blemishes. Lemon juice is applied frequently to skin blemishes and discolorations.

JEWELWEED

Botanical Name: *Impatiens biflora*
Common Names: Spotted Jewels, Spotted Touch-Me-Not, Wild Balsam

Jewelweed is widely distributed over North America, Africa, the Asiatic mountains, and the East Indies. It is a tall plant growing in damp, rich soil along streams and similar damp locations. The slipper-shaped orange-yellow flowers are covered with dark spots and bloom from July to September. When ripe, the pods discharge the seeds under the slightest disturbance, scattering them widely.

Remedial Use

Jewelweed was well known and used by the American Indians as an effective treatment for poison oak and poison ivy. Many people living in the country who are familiar with its use also claim it is highly effective. The fresh plant stems and leaves are mashed, and the juice is rubbed on the skin. It is also considered an excellent preventive by applying the juice on the exposed skin before going into areas of the country in which poison oak and poison ivy may be growing. The juice is also said to remove warts and corns and to cure ringworm.

The jewelweed plant may be obtained from a garden nursery, or the liquid extract or decoction can be used instead, applied to the skin as a wash.

Case Study

Mr. R. S. writes: "I love to hike in the country but have always been extremely susceptible to poison oak, which has caused me many sleepless nights and lost work days. Even if the poison oak plant was quite a distance away and the wind was blowing past it in my direction, I became infected. Doctors prescribed cortisone, which helped but gave me bad side effects.

"I found that the terrible itching could be immediately relieved by running very hot water, as hot as I could stand it, on the infected areas of my skin, but the relief, as welcome as it was, lasted only a very few minutes.

"Then one day I came across an article about herbs which were used by the Indians. It said that the Omahas applied the juice from the crushed leaves of a plant called jewelweed for skin rashes and eczema, and that the Potawatomis used the same plant to treat poison oak, poison ivy, and nettle stings.

"I figured that since the Indians lived close to Nature, they knew what they were talking about. So the next time I contracted poison oak I immediately purchased a jewelweed plant and rubbed the juice over the affected parts of my skin. It worked! What a Godsend!

"I have since discovered that making a decoction of jewelweed and rubbing it on my skin before going on a hike prevents me from getting poison oak even if I accidentally brush against the plant. Others should know about this remarkable remedy."

BLACKSTRAP MOLASSES

Some cases of dermatitis, eczema, and psoriasis have reportedly responded to the therapeutic power of blackstrap molasses. Cyril Scott reports: "Experience over a period of nine years has proved that the molasses treatment is a rational and natural scientific method of curing skin diseases. These include dry eczema, weeping eczema, and even some types of psoriasis, when not due to an emotional disturbance."

Scott mentions the case of Mr. L., whose hands were very red and swollen with dermatitis. The man was induced to soak his hands frequently in water to which some molasses had been added and to take molasses several times a day. Scott reports: "The cure was complete in six weeks."[1]

ECHINACEA

Botanical Name: *Echinacea angustifolia—Echinacea purpurea*
Common Names: Coneflower, Purple Coneflower

Echinacea refers to both *Echinacea angustifolia* and *Echinacea purpurea*. They have similar properties and are classed as alterative (blood purifier) and antiseptic.

Echinacea enhances the defensive powers of the body against infection and is used for various toxic conditions such as bacterial and viral infections, skin eruptions, eczema, acne, psoriasis, insect stings, poison ivy, and poison oak. It is available on the market in the form of tinctures, tablets, extracts, and ointments and is often combined with other similar herbs. Directions for its use are included with the various products.

Echinacin™ is derived from the fresh plant juice of *Echinacea purpurea*. It has been effectively employed in Europe as a supportive measure for dermatological disorders and is sold in the U.S. under the name Echinace™.

Case Studies

"In January of this year I attracted an allergy which had me covered all around the neck, shoulders, and arms in a scarlet-quilt pattern rash. Parts of me looked and felt as though I had been having fun and games in a beehive. In short, I was an unholy mess. I never knew itching and burning could be so vicious.

"For five weeks I took the doctor's 10 tablets a day. For a number of weeks following this, there was a switch to antibiotics and then a spell on cortisone tablets.

"The doctor again put me on 'allergy-chasers' and said there was little more he could do; but he was good enough to make an appointment for me to see a skin specialist. After months of disappointments, I decided to cancel that appointment and instead decided to take echinacea tablets. I have not had a single spot since the first week I started taking them. Now you can't see where those ugly spots have been.

"Incidentally, a dark blue bruisy patch stemming from my right inner ankle and rising to the knee in a vivid etching of red and blue, which I have been conscious of for two years, has practically disappeared." —Mrs. L. N.

"I wish to tell you the benefit brought to me by echinacea tablets. I had been troubled with eczema for some time, and an ointment had been prescribed by my doctor. The irritation was wretched, but after taking echinacea for a few days, the irritation disappeared entirely. I am truly thankful." —Miss M. M.

"Last year I had four bottles of echinacea. It may be too soon to boast, but at the time of writing, my rash and itches which I have had for several years, in spite of various treatments, have almost completely vanished." —C. T. W.

"Some months ago my friend gave me a bottle of echinacea extract and suggested I try it. What a wonderful effect it has had in clearing up a flaky skin condition I have been troubled with for more than 18 months. This is the first preparation I have tried that has done me any good." —Mrs. E. S.

European Medical Studies on Echinacin™

Dr. Gaertner employed Echinacin™ extract in treating patients with psoriasis.[2] They were given a dose of 30 to 50 drops of the extract three times daily, along with conventional topical therapy. Definite remissions occurred in 90% of the cases, sometimes with complete disappearance of the skin's lesions. However, the treatment was ineffective when the disease involved large areas. For most patients, the therapy extended over a period of 9 to 18 months.

Echinacin™ has also been used with success when applied locally. A large-scale trial[3] (not performed in hospitals) demonstrated that Echinacin™ ointment is effective for numerous skin conditions. Five hundred and thirty-eight medical specialists participated in the study. The trial involved 4,598 patients with inflammatory skin conditions such as dermatitis, abscesses, folliculitis (inflammation of the hair follicles of the skin), myoderma (a pustular condition of the skin which may be in the form of small pimples, abscesses, or carbuncles); wounds; varicose ulcers of the legs; herpes simplex; and various forms of eczema.

The overall rate of success, 85%, was highly significant. In more than 90% of all cases of herpes simplex, burns, and skin wounds, the lesions disappeared within one week. On the average, symptoms were relieved within four days. Eighty-three percent of the patients with eczema improved, as did 71% of those troubled with varicose ulceration of the leg. For most conditions, the failure rate was only 10%, except for leg ulcers, which was 17%.

Smaller tests have shown, too, that Echinacin™ ointment works exceptionally well for the treatment of wounds, as it is free from side effects as compared with ointments containing steroids or antibiotics.[4]

SLIPPERY ELM

Botanical Name: *Ulmus fulva*
Common Names: American Elm, Sweet Elm, Rock Elm, Moose Elm, Red Elm

This deciduous tree grows abundantly in various areas of North America. It has very rough branches and rough down leaves of a deep yellowish-orange color. During March and April, the tree bears clusters of tiny, stalkless flowers.

Remedial Uses

Slippery Elm is classed as demulcent, nutritive, emollient, pectoral, and diuretic. The finely powdered bark has long been valued not only as a soothing internal healer for irritations of the lungs, stomach, and intestines but also as a poultice for all inflamed surfaces, skin diseases, chilblains, abscesses, warts, ulcers, etc. The poultice quickly disperses inflammation and draws out impurities.

The poultice is prepared by mixing slippery elm powder with hot water to form the required consistency. This is spread on a soft cotton cloth and applied to the affected area.

Case Study

One man reported that for 30 years he had a wart on the palm of his hand which gave him no trouble until suddenly it grew larger and became inflamed. A chiropodist friend recommended having it surgically removed at a hospital, but the man's wife suggested he try slippery elm instead, and he agreed. He writes: "I made this (slippery elm powder) into a 'blob' which I placed on the wart, and I kept it covered with a bit of lint or cotton wool secured with two cross-pieces of half-inch bandage. I changed the whole thing roughly every other day for about four weeks, by which time the inflammation had gone and the wart had shrunk to the size of a pin's head. I then changed over from slippery elm to a tiny slice of lemon peel, affixed in the same way. In about another week the tiny black wart was loose in its moorings, and a gentle sideways scrape of my fingernail completely detached it. I subsequently gave the site of the wart a dab or two of lemon juice, and there is now a perfect healing."

SOYBEAN LECITHIN

There have been many reports on the value of lecithin for treating psoriasis, the noninfectious skin disease symptomized by patchy areas, often on the elbows, hands, knees, and scalp. In this condition the areas are pink or red and covered with dry, silvery scales, which may vary from a thick layer to a large mass.

In her book,[5] nutritionalist Adele Davis reported:

> The eczema-like skin condition psoriasis appears to result from faulty utilization of fats. People with this abnormality usually have excessive amounts of cholesterol in their skin and blood, and by the time their blood cholesterol has been reduced to normal their psoriasis clears up. When 254 patients with psoriasis were given 4 to 8 tablespoons of lecithin daily no new eruptions occurred after the first week and even the most severe cases recovered within five months. Psoriasis has also been helped by vitamins A and B6. I recommend only 3 tablespoons of granular lecithin daily with every nutrient to help the liver produce its own lecithin.

The successful treatment of psoriasis with lecithin was also reported by Doctors Beatrice Kesten and Paul Groves of the Department of Dermatology at the Columbia-Presbyterian Medical Center. Two hundred and thirty-five patients were placed on a lecithin and low fat diet. Because of the restricted diet, vitamin supplements were also administered, but the physicians were convinced that the soybean lecithin was the agent responsible for the beneficial effects on the condition of psoriasis.

Of the 235 patients, 155 were considered adequately treated. The rest either refused to cooperate or abandoned the program before conclusions could be reached. Only 37 of those who followed the procedure experienced no improvement. Twenty-three became well after one year of treatment and three years of observation. Twenty-nine were highly pleased that their psoriasis was being controlled. The remaining 66 subjects showed some improvement but required special ointments in addition to taking lecithin.

Individual Case Histories

One woman had suffered with psoriasis on her arms and hands for over 20 years. After using lecithin in her diet, she reported that her skin became clean, smooth, and clear of scabs. She found that if she discontinued the lecithin she experienced a recurrence of psoriasis. In another case, a woman complained of psoriasis on her elbows and knees, which were red, itchy, and even bleeding when the scales were removed. A short time after taking lecithin capsules, the condition cleared up.

Mrs. T. S. writes: "My brother had a serious case of psoriasis for three years. It was in his scalp, and on his face, arms and legs. Doctors were unable to cure him. My daughter heard about lecithin and told him to take one capsule of 1,200 milligrams of liquid lecithin twice daily. Several weeks later the psoriasis began to clear, and after another month it was completely gone and hasn't returned. This has been like a miracle. He now takes just one lecithin capsule every day to prevent the condition from coming back."

Lecithin for Diaper Rash

A woman's three-month-old infant daughter was affected by diaper rash. The mother washed the baby after every diaper change, but the rash persisted. She was advised by the pediatrician to use a medicated ointment, but it only made the rash worse. She says: "My neighbor told me to get some capsules of 1,200 milligrams of liquid lecithin from a health food store and to cut the end off the capsule, squeeze the oil out, and smear it on the baby's bottom. The next time the baby wet, I changed and washed her and then applied the thick lecithin oil. After the next diaper change, the rash showed some improvement.

Encouraged, I continued the procedure with each diaper change, and in just a few days the rash could no longer be seen. To prevent any return of the problem, I apply lecithin on her bottom once a day after her bath, and there has been no further trouble.

"I have passed my experience on to many others whose babies were bothered with diaper rash and have not heard of a single failure when lecithin oil was applied."

PROPOLIS

Propolis, which was discussed in detail in chapter 7, has been used with good effect for the following skin conditions.

Acne
Propolis tincture applied several times daily reportedly promotes rapid healing and forms an invisible coating which protects against renewed infection.

Corns
Propolis cream is applied each night and morning, and the corn is covered with a small gauze bandage.

Dry Eczema
One propolis capsule is taken twice daily for a few days, and then propolis cream is applied once a day. This treatment is used only for dry eczema, as it will aggravate wet eczema.

Warts
Propolis tincture is applied once or twice every day.

Mouth Ulcers
A dab of propolis tincture is applied to the ulcer two or three times daily or propolis lozenges may be used. In addition, propolis cream or tincture is applied to the affected area at night before retiring.

Shingles
One propolis capsule is taken between meals twice daily.

Medical Experiences with Propolis

At a symposium in Yugoslavia, Dr. Franz Feiks reported treating 21 cases of shingles with dressings of propolis tincture. The pain disappeared in 48 hours in all 21 cases and did not return. In 19 patients, the skin sores were completely healed.

In Austria, Dr. Edith Lauda wanted to establish whether propolis had an antibacterial effect on human skin. Fifty-nine patients with different types of acne, which they had suffered with for several years, were treated with propolis tincture and propolis ointment. Twenty-five of the cases of acne simplex were cured at home within seven days. Others affected with more severe forms of acne were healed within three weeks. Along with home treatment, these cases had only three weekly treatments at the clinic.

One patient with acne conglobata had been treated by a number of dermatologists for 30 years without success. After just two propolis treatments her skin was free of inflammation, and only very small marks were visible.

Another remarkable case was that of a 40-year-old patient who had tried every possible treatment for acne pustulosa which covered her entire face. In two weeks the acne had completely disappeared after she treated herself at home with propolis tincture and ointment.

Many women suffer from vaginal *Candida albicans,*a fungus infection. Some medics blame the free lifestyle among the young and the use of the pill, which creates a suitable environment for the Candida fungus. However, a propolis pessary is reportedly achieving curative results. Studies to prove this began with a team of four doctors headed by Dr. Ishida of the Tokohu University School of Medicine in Japan.

Later these studies were carried on by Doctors Cizmarik and Troupl of the University of Bratislava, Czechoslovakia who tested propolis with very good results on a whole range of fungi. They continued their tests and concluded that propolis is remarkably effective for all fungal infections of the skin and body.[6]

MYRRH

Botanical Name: *Balsamodendron myrrh*
Common Names: Myrrha, Mira

Myrrh is a shrub or tree native to Arabia, Abyssinia, and other countries bordering the Red Sea. It is quite low and branchy with whitish-grey bark and bears fruit about the size of a pea. The juice flows naturally from the bark, forming soft, reddish-brown drops or tears which gradually harden and form the medicinal gum myrrh. These drops vary in size from that of a small grain to as large as a walnut. They powder readily, giving off a pleasant balsamic fragrance.

Early Uses

Myrrh is one of humankind's oldest favorites among the botanicals and has been used in perfumes, ointments, scented candles, and incense. It was one of the ingredients of the oil with which the Jews anointed the Tabernacle, the Ark, the altars, and sacred vessels. The purification of women as ordained by Jewish law lasted 12 months, the first six being accompanied with oil of myrrh.

Of the Three Wise Men, believed to be members of the priestly caste of Persia, one offered a gift of myrrh to the Infant Jesus, as it was valued on par with gold.

Modern Uses

Medicinally, tincture of myrrh is applied full strength as an antiseptic to minor skin irritations and cold sores. As a mouthwash, 1/2 teaspoon of the tincture in a glass of warm water is very soothing and healing for troublesome mouth ulcers, canker sores, and denture-irritated gums or when gums are sore from rough brushing or sensitive dental work. Its lovely fragrance also refreshes and sweetens the breath.

APPLE CIDER VINEGAR

Apple cider vinegar is used for treating numerous skin problems including athlete's foot, a burning, itching fungus infection caused by the presence of a tiny microorganism. There are several things which can contribute to getting the infection: profuse sweating of the feet; uncleanliness; friction of the stockings and shoes against the feet; direct contact with the fungus (for example, stepping into a shower that has been used by someone who has athlete's foot).

Because of its contagious nature, this fungus infection can spread to other areas of the body, such as the face and hands, due to contact with the original site.

To remedy the condition, the feet are washed thoroughly but lightly with a soft brush and mild soap and warm water. The washing is continued for about 5 or 10 minutes, working up a good lather, and then the feet are rinsed and patted dry. Apple cider vinegar is then applied to the feet, including areas in between the toes.

A fresh towel should be used for drying the feet after each foot bath, and the stockings should be changed every day. To prevent reinfection, the soiled socks and towels should be boiled for 15 minutes.

Other Uses of Apple Cider Vinegar

For poison ivy, equal parts of apple cider vinegar and water are dabbed on the affected parts of the skin and allowed to dry; in conditions of shingles the vinegar is used straight from the bottle to the troublesome area four times a day, and if possible two or three times during the night; for ringworm of the scalp it is applied to the affected area with the fingers. Impetigo, a highly contagious infection of the skin, usually clears up in a few days with applications of the vinegar six times daily, at intervals.

Nature's Deodorant

Apple cider vinegar is an excellent underarm deodorant when used directly after bathing. The strong vinegar aroma fades quickly in just a few moments after it has been applied. This simple, inexpensive natural deodorant lasts for many hours. It does not stop the normal discharge of perspiration (a healthy function which releases toxins from the body) but thoroughly eliminates the disagreeable underarm odor.

For those who wish to do so, the vinegar may be scented with one or more fragrant herbs (e.g., lavender flowers, rosemary, sweet woodruff, chamomile, orris root). It is prepared by bringing 1 pint of apple cider vinegar to a boil. As soon as it boils, 1 ounce of the herb or herbs is added, and the burner is immediately turned off. The container is covered with a lid, and the preparation is allowed to stand until cold. It is then strained and bottled for use.

CASTOR OIL

Botanical Name: *Ricinus communis*
Common Name: Palma Christi

Brown spots, often called liver spots, which appear on the hands and face of older people, have been removed by applications of castor oil. Dr. Jarvis tells of a patient who had about a dozen such spots on the backs of his hands. The patient followed the doctor's instructions to apply castor oil to the spots night and morning, rubbing it well into the skin. By the end of one month, they could no longer be seen.[7]

Dr. Jarvis also reports on the effectiveness of castor oil in removing brown moles from the skin. He mentions the case of a woman who had a mole about the size of her little fingernail in the center of her cheek. The dark mole could be seen through her makeup, and she told the doctor that it had been there for as long as she could remember. She was advised to rub castor oil on the area after removing her makeup each night, wiping off the excess oil as she was ready to get into bed. At the end of the week, the color of the mole had started to fade. Three weeks later it had completely disappeared. Dr. Jarvis says, "I could see a smooth place where the mole had been, but its color was that of the surrounding skin."[8]

William A. McGarey, M.D., reports:[9] "One of my patients had a pigmented mole in the inguinal area. After I discovered it, she did not show up again for some time. When I saw her next she told me she had applied castor oil to the mole for two weeks, and it disappeared. I checked, and it was no longer there."

Plantar Warts

A wart which develops on the bottom of the foot is called a plantar wart. This is more deeply imbedded than warts that appear on other areas of the body.

For dispersing plantar warts, a pad of cotton saturated with castor oil is bound on the wart at bedtime. The treatment is repeated nightly until results are achieved (generally in about three or four weeks).

Sore Feet, Calluses, Corns, and Bunions

Rubbing castor oil on the feet at bedtime and allowing it to remain on all night reduces callus build-up and softens corns and dry, cracked skin. A pair of cotton socks is worn to protect the sheets. After a few nights the feet will feel smooth, soft, and comfortable and will stay warm on cold nights.

Dr. McGarey mentions the case of a women who treated a bunion on her big toe by rubbing it with castor oil three times daily and sleeping with a pad placed over it at night, Dr. McGarey says: "In three weeks, the swelling was gone. Whenever it starts to flare up again, she treats it the same way with the same results."[10]

Chapped Lips and Mouth Ulcers

To relieve the soreness of mouth ulcers, Mrs. A. R. smears them with just a light touch of castor oil. She explains: "Although it does not prevent them, it takes the pain right out of them—as if by a miracle. I can eat and smile—two things which are difficult when you have mouth ulcers the size of half a pea. So many other things have been tried, and benefits have not lasted. But castor oil really works."

Applied to the lips, castor oil helps protect them against chapping, drying, or cracking on cold, windy days.

Napkin Dermatosis

The affected parts are first bathed with warm chamomile tea and then patted dry. Castor oil is then applied to the troublesome areas.

Sties and Warts

Sties and warts have been effectively eliminated with applications of castor oil. Consider the following cases:

"With me, a sty lasts only a few days when anointed with castor oil. A friend of mine had a bad sty. I advised her to use the oil. She did so. She was amazed at its disappearance within two or three days. She passed the information to another woman whose eyes were troubled in this way, and that lady, too, was surprised at an almost immediate response." —R. V.

"Over 50 years ago, my mother had large warts covering her hands. Having a persevering nature, she tried many remedies. Then she tried castor oil. This was applied several times during the day. They started to diminish. Finally, 'All clear'." —G. O.

"I was rather worried about a little white wart on my eyelid. The doctor told me, 'You have it to stay.' After having tried quite a few remedies, it looked alive as ever. So I decided to have a try with castor oil. For about three months, twice a day, I applied it and it got smaller and smaller. Another three weeks it was gone and has not returned. That was about a year ago." —Miss M. R.

A correspondent writes: "Last summer a friend told me her son was going on a holiday on the Continent the next day and was very distressed because he had a large patch of warts on his face. They had been damaged by shaving and were wet and oozing. His doctor suggested an electric razor.

"I looked up some references in my natural health books and told him to rub castor oil well into the warts, night and morning (about 20 rubs each time) and to take a course of vitamin A (halibut liver oil capsules). This he did. Within 15 days the trouble had completely cleared. They were surprised, as his mother said he had been troubled by warts since childhood."

SUMMARY

1. Certain herbs and herbal products provide natural and effective ways of coping with many skin disorders.

2. The common lemon may be used in a number of ways for problems involving the skin.

3. Some cases of dermatitis, eczema, and psoriasis have reportedly responded to the therapeutic power of blackstrap molasses.

4. The jewelweed plant, a time-tested remedy for poison oak and poison ivy, can usually be obtained from a garden nursery.

5. Echinacea, classed as a blood purifier and antiseptic, is available on the market in the form of tablets, extracts, tinctures, and ointments for use in treating certain skin conditions.

6. Echinacin^{TM} has been effectively employed in Europe as a supportive measure for dermatological problems and is sold in the U.S, under the name Echinace^{TM}.

7. Poultices of slippery elm quickly disperse surface inflammation and draw out impurities from the skin.

8. Soybean lecithin has proved effective in some cases of psoriasis.

9. Propolis has been used with success for a wide range of skin disorders.

10. Anyone allergic to propolis should not use it in any form.

11. Tincture of myrrh may be applied straight from the bottle to cold sores and skin irritations; diluted, it produces a healing effect on mouth ulcers, canker sores, and denture-irritated gums.

12. Apple cider vinegar has effectively treated numerous skin problems including the fungus infection of athlete's foot, which can spread to other areas of the body due to contact with the original site.

13. Applications of castor oil have eliminated many trouble-some skin conditions.

ENDNOTES

1. *Crude Black Molasses* (Wellingborough, England: Athene Pub. Co., Ltd.).

2. *Nonspecific Enchancement of Intrinsic Resistance to Infection by Echinacin.* K. Ch. Schimmel and G. T. Werner (Ther. d Gegnw., 1981).

3. Ibid.

4. Ibid.

5. *Let's Get Well* (New York: Harcourt, Brace & World, Inc.)

6. Maurice Hanssen, *The Healing Power of Pollen and Other Products From the Bee Hive* (Wellingborough, Northhamptonshire, England: Thorsons Pub., Ltd.).

7. D. C. Jarvis, M.D., *Folk Medicine* (New York: Henry Holt & Co.).

8. Ibid.

9. Director, Medical Research Division, The Edgar Cayce Fdn., Phoenix, Ariz.

10. Ibid.

C H A P T E R   1 0

HERB REMEDIES
FOR RESPIRATORY
AILMENTS

Coughing is the most commonly occurring respiratory symptom and is often an expression of some disease in the lungs or the bronchial tubes. It indicates Nature's effort to expel excessive mucus or irritating material from the air passages. If the deposits are deep-seated and stubborn, the cough may persist. It may also persist when the lungs are irritated by smoke or infection, even though there is no material to eject.

A dry cough occurs when there is congestion in the lining of the bronchial tubes as in the early stages of acute bronchitis. Coughs may also result from other causes, such as an enlarged heart, or in some cases may be of a nervous origin.

The common cold is an inflammation of the membrane lining of the nose and upper air passage caused by a virus, but secondary infection with bacteria often follows.

The usual symptoms are headache, chills, sneezing, coughing, loss of appetite, a slight rise in temperature, and nasal congestion followed by a watery discharge which gradually becomes thick and purulent. Sometimes the inflammation spreads to the throat, causing soreness and difficulty in swallowing. When the larynx is affected, the voice becomes hoarse, and if the infection spreads further down into the chest, bronchitis or laryngitis may develop.

Other Types of Pulmonary Ailments

There are many other infections or ailments of the respiratory tract which cause considerable suffering. The following are a few of the most common.

153

Influenza. Influenza is an acute infectious disease which attacks the air passages and may give rise to serious complications. The infection is symptomized by fever, severe headache, chills, sore throat, coughing, sneezing, pains in the muscles, and watering of the eyes and nose. The onset of the symptoms is generally rapid, from one to three days. Temperature may rise suddenly to 100 to 104 degrees. The infection often occurs in epidemics and is spread by droplets from coughing and sneezing.

Asthma. The term *asthma* generally refers to bronchial asthma, a condition resulting from an allergic reaction in the small chest tubes, the bronchioles. It is symptomized by wheezing, shortness of breath, coughing, mucous sputum, and difficulty in exhaling air. The paroxysms of severe shortness of breath and the wheezing result from temporary narrowing of the bronchi by mucosal swelling, muscle spasms, and thick, fluid secretion. Dr. Hong-Yen Hsu explains, "Some people think that in an asthmatic attack there is difficulty in inhalation. This is wrong; the difficulty lies in exhalation. Because the exchange between CO_2 and O_2 in the lungs cannot be carried out smoothly there is a lack of oxygen; thus many patients need to open the windows of their rooms."[1]

An asthmatic attack generally occurs at night but may sometimes occur during the day and may last a few minutes to several hours. It often occurs at the same time each night for several weeks and may disappear for a period of weeks or months. During an attack, the sufferer usually hunches the shoulders in an attempt to facilitate breathing.

Bronchitis. Inflammation of the bronchial tubes is known as bronchitis. It can be acute or chronic. Acute conditions are symptomized by coughing, expectoration, hoarseness, chills, fever and throat irritation. Once the disease is firmly established, it becomes chronic and generally affects men more than women. The main symptoms are shortness of breath on exertion, severe exhausting cough, and "moist rales" (whistling wheezes in the chest when exhaling); sputum may be profuse and watery, or scant and tenuous, and may be streaked with blood. Exposure to wet, damp weather worsens the condition, which is why medics advise people with bronchitis to live in a warm, dry climate if possible.

Emphysema. In normal breathing, the lungs quickly spring back to their normal shape after expansion by inhalation, In emphysema, elasticity is lost and the lungs become permanently expanded. The condition differs from chronic bronchitis because it destroys the walls or the air sacs.

The most characteristic symptom of the disease is shortness of breath, At first, breathlessness is present only on exertion, but in advanced cases it is constant. Through lack of oxygen, muscles weaken. The rate of breathing may increase 14 to 30 times per minute. Coughing and clearing the throat are almost invariably constant. The condition becomes extremely severe during an attack of asthma or bronchitis, which often occur in the late stages of the disease.

Pleurisy. This is a condition in which the lining of the pleural membrane and its reflection over the inner surfaces of the chest wall become inflamed. It is symptomized by pain which is aggravated by deep breathing, coughing, or sneezing. Most cases are caused by chill from exposure to cold winds and damp, wet weather.

Hay Fever. Hay fever is an allergic disease caused by sensitivity to plant pollen and other irritating particles. An attack causes sneezing, watery, itching eyes, and runny nose. The nasal mucous membrane is inflamed and swollen.

HERBS FOR COPING WITH RESPIRATORY DISEASES

Along with using any of the following herb remedies, a healthy diet should be adopted with emphasis on fresh fruits and vegetables. Proper rest, fresh air, keeping the bowels open, and the daily use of supplements are also important.

COLTSFOOT

Botanical Name: *Tussilago farfara*
Common Name: Coughwort, Horsehoof, Foalwort, Calves Foot

This perennial herb is native to India but is common in many lands. It reaches from one-half to 1 foot high, prefers clay soil, and bears large, daisy-type bright yellow flowers, one to each stalk, Its hoof-shaped leaves do not appear until after the flowers have withered.

Early Uses

The botanical name of coltsfoot *tussilago* means "cough dispeller," indicating the herb's reputation as a remedy for lung problems. Dioscorides, Pliny, and Galen recommended smoking the leaves of coltsfoot for coughs, colds, bronchitis, and asthma. Culpeper, the herbalist of the early seventeenth century, advised using the fresh leaves, juice, or syrup for a "bad dry cough or wheezing and shortness of breath."

At one time coltsfoot was considered so valuable in France as a medicine that it became an insignia of apothecary shops.

Modern Uses

Coltsfoot is classed as expectorant, pectoral, and demulcent. A decoction of the herb is used in lung and bronchial ailments for loosening mucus and relieving irritation and persistent coughing. Its influence is more apparent, however, when inflammation is present, probably because it contains large amounts of mucilage, which protects the lungs.

The decoction is prepared with 1 ounce of the herb to 1-1/2 pints of water brought to a boil, simmered slowly down to 1 pint, and then strained. One teacup sweetened with honey is taken three times a day.

To relieve congestion and difficult breathing in conditions of bronchitis, the following formula is employed:

> Coltsfoot: 1 oz.
>
> Elecampane: 1/2 oz.
>
> Marshmallow: 1/4 oz.

Horehound, hyssop, and violet leaves add power to coltsfoot in relieving the persistent cough of weaker persons or those who have been exhausted by the debility of chronic catarrh. The decoction is prepared by mixing together 1 ounce each of coltsfoot, hyssop, horehound, and violet leaves. One half of the mixture is simmered in 2 pints of water down to 1-1/2 pints and then strained. This is taken frequently in teacupful doses sweetened with honey.

ELEUTHERO

Botanical Name: *Eleutherococcus senticosis*
Common Names: Siberian Ginseng, Touch-Me-Not

Data accumulated by Soviet research teams has shown that eleuthero has an antiinfluenzal effect. A group of young men in the Primorya region were given eleuthero extract every other day during the month of March. The influenza and acute respiratory diseases (ARD) were reduced from 17% to 12.7% as compared to a control group that did not take the extract.[2]

In another study, about 1,000 workers at the Norilisk mining and smelter plant took eleuthero extract daily for two months. The influenza and ARD incidence decreased almost 2.4 times in contrast to the same number of workers at the same shop working under the same conditions but who were not given the extract.[3]

YERBA SANTA

Botanical Name: *Eriodictyon californicum*
Common Names: Holy Herb, Consumptive Weed, Mountain Balm

This aromatic evergreen shrub reaching from 3 to 7 feet high is indigenous to the mountains of California, Oregon and northern Mexico. The glutinous leaves, which are 3 to 4 inches in length, grow alternately on the smooth stem, which exudes a peculiar resinous substance. Flowers are blue or whitish, appearing in clusters at the top of the plant.

Early Uses

Yerba Santa was highly valued by the Indians for treating respiratory complaints. The leaves were smoked or chewed for relieving asthma, and as a remedy for colds and catarrh a tea was prepared from the leaves and taken daily for several days.

The remedial use of Yerba Santa was soon adopted by the early settlers and Spanish missionaries, who considered it of special value in chronic inflammation of the bronchial tubes. It was also employed as a treatment for consumption.

Modern Uses

Yerba Santa is classed as expectorant, febrifuge, and antispasmodic. It is used for treating the spasm of asthma and for colds, catarrh, chronic bronchitis, laryngitis, and throat irritation. It is also used to reduce fever.

The infusion is prepared by placing 1 teaspoonful of the leaves in a cup of boiling water and allowing it to stand for half an hour. It is then strained, and one-half cupful is taken either hot or cold at night when retiring, or a large mouthful three times a day. A total of 1 or 2 cups may be taken daily.

If the tincture is used instead, 10 to 30 drops are taken in a small glass of water once or twice a day.

ICELAND MOSS

Botanical Name: *Cetraria islandica*
Common Names: Cetraria, Iceland Lichen

This is not actually a moss but a lichen, native to Britain and northern countries of Europe, especially Iceland. It is also found in certain northern areas of North America. The thallus, or body of the plant, is smooth, grey, or light olive brown, branching about 2 to 4 inches high, terminating in spreading, flattened lobes. The under surface is paler with minute, depressed white spots.

Medicinal Uses

Iceland moss is classed as demulcent, tonic, and nutritive. Decoctions or tablets made from the plant are highly recommended by herbalists for treating colds, hoarseness, and bronchitis.

The decoction is prepared by placing 1 tablespoon of Iceland moss with 1-1/2 cups of cold milk in a Pyrex® or enamel pot. The container is covered with a lid, and the beverage is brought to a boil. After it has boiled slowly for three or four minutes, it is removed from the burner and strained. The decoction is kept covered with a lid, allowed to stand for three minutes, and then reheated and drank as hot as possible at bedtime.

Some Impressive Case Studies

"I must tell you that since taking Iceland Moss tablets my friend who suffers from emphysema has found great relief. Especially with bronchitis last winter. He was very ill when I sent for Iceland Moss tablets; now we both firmly believe they are working wonders."[4] —Miss C. C.

"I am happy to report that a hot beverage of Iceland moss cured my attack of bronchitis. Not only that, but I told a coworker about it who had a nasty cough she couldn't seem to get rid of in spite of medical treatment. Was she ever delighted when her coughing spells cleared up after taking my Iceland moss remedy." —L. T. R.

"About a year ago I had a dreadful cold in my chest. After lots of antibiotics given by my doctor I was still as bad as ever. In desperation I rang an Herbalist who very kindly advised me to take Iceland Moss tablets, every so many hours through the day and two rose hip capsules morning and evening. This I did. It worked like magic. In no time I was better. In about a week or ten days completely well. I always keep Iceland Moss and rose hip by me, and have been able to help my friends."[5] —A. S.

"Since my daughter began taking Iceland moss in the form of tablets, she has had neither a cough or a cold. That is remarkable, because she is very susceptible to both." —Mrs. S. L.

GINKGO TREE

Botanical Name: *Ginkgo biloba*
Common Name: Ginkgo

Dr. Joachim H. Volkner, a nose, ear, and throat specialist in Berlin found that if a person suffering from a common cold inhales an essence prepared from ginkgo leaves, the cold will get better. Results in treating 224 people who used the essence were reported to be excellent, as the inflamed areas "healed immediately."

Dr. Volkner explained how the treatment works. When someone has a cold, the cells of the mucous membranes are damaged and unable to store moisture. The efficiency of the cell walls becomes impaired due to substances in the cell pressing against these walls. Inhaling the essence of ginkgo apparently forces these components of the cell back into its interior. Dr. Volkner states, "The microbes which have collected die off, and very shortly after inhalation (of the ginkgo essence) they completely disappear."[6]

GARLIC

Botanical Name: *Allium sativum*
Common Names: Clove Garlic, Poor Man's Treacle

Garlic is a miracle remedy that can help prevent or heal numerous respiratory ailments. In the 1960s tons of garlic were used in Russia to bring a halt to a massive flu epidemic. People were advised to consume more garlic as a means of protection against the disease. If you feel a sore throat or cold coming on, researchers at Brigham Young University[7] advise eating some garlic or onions. James North, chief of microbiology at BYU, says, "If you do it early enough you may not even get sick." The laboratory studies demonstrated that among other things garlic extract can destroy with almost 100% effectiveness human rhinovirus—which causes colds; parainfluenza 3—a common respiratory and flu virus; and herpes simplex 1—which causes fever blisters. North says that their studies have established that garlic "kills on contact with the virus."

Home Remedies Using Garlic

Here are a few of many examples in which garlic is used as a domestic remedy for treating certain respiratory disorders:

- Garlic, chopped finely and added to soups, salads, and vegetable juices, is used for the relief of colds, asthma, bronchitis, nasal congestion, pleurisy, and seizures of prolonged sneezing.

- Mucus accumulates during sleep, and this is where two or three garlic capsules at bedtime can prove helpful.

- Three garlic tablets taken in the morning and three at night are used for sinus trouble and hay fever.

- For influenza, three to four capsules of Kyolic® Formula 103, containing garlic extract powder, vitamin C, astragalus, and calcium lactate, are taken every hour until the condition improves. Rest and drinking plenty of liquids are also important in conditions of influenza.

- A teaspoon of freshly expressed garlic juice well mixed with honey, and a teaspoonful taken at repeated intervals, is used for the relief of colds, cough, bronchitis, asthma, and sore throat.

- To relieve sinusitis, Kyolic® liquid garlic is diluted with water and used as nose drops three times a day for several days. In addition, four Kyolic® garlic capsules are taken three times daily.

- One teaspoon of Kyolic® liquid garlic diluted with water is used as a gargle for sore throat and tonsillitis.

- For allergic rhinitis (hay fever) four to six capsules of Kyolic® Formula 102 are taken daily. This priceless formula is a harmless alternative to injections and drugs.

Whooping Cough. The use of herbal medications applied to the feet was a common practice in the days of our grandparents. There is a lot to be said for it, as poulticing the feet with pulped garlic has proved successful in eliminating toxins of some childhood diseases, including whooping cough.

To prepare the remedy, small sections of garlic cloves are pulped or chopped fine, enough to make each poultice about 1/4 inch thick to cover the bottom of each foot. The garlic is spread evenly on a thin piece of soft cloth, and another thin piece of cloth is placed over the garlic.

Before applying the poultice, the bottoms of the feet are greased with Vaseline®. If the poultice is placed directly on the skin, the garlic is apt to cause blisters. The poultice is placed on another thin cloth suitable for binding it on overnight, and each foot is then covered with a clean sock.

In the morning the poultices are removed, and fresh ones prepared again at night and used as before. Garlic can be detected on the patient's breath the next morning after application, attesting to its absorption.

The poulticing is continued nightly until results are achieved.

This same treatment also works very well for anyone having a hard night cough.

Case Studies Demonstrate Garlic's Healing Power

In his writings, medical herbalist J. H. Oliver presents a slightly different method of poulticing the feet for treating whooping cough, and he also mentions an impressive case history:[8]

> *Whooping Cough*—Put the sufferer to bed. Place a layer of lint on the sole of the foot and fasten. Crush some garlic pods to a pulp and spread it all over the layers of lint. *It must not touch the skin.* Cover with oiled silk and fasten.
>
> A typical case of faith in our methods and skepticism on the part of others was shown when a father returned home and found his four children down with a severe attack of whooping cough. He put them to bed and proceeded to treat them as advised above. Everybody laughed at him. The idea of treating the soles of the feet for a trouble in the chest seemed to the skeptics the last word in absurdity— especially *such* a treatment. However, the laugh was soon on the other side, for they all had a peaceful night, and in the morning the whooping cough had gone, and didn't return. Many similar successes could be described—much to the discomfiture of the skeptics. The cures have been so swift that the usually unbelieving Thomases in most cases refuse to believe that the attacks were whooping cough at all. They seemed to be obsessed with the idea that it must "run its course."

A correspondent writes: "You may be interested in this. When I was a young child, I had whooping cough. When I was over the worst of it, the doctor told my mother to put garlic in my shoes. He said he knew it was a strange thing to do, but if people only knew, a lot of toxins can be drawn out of the body through the feet. So I walked on garlic, and suffered no after effects of the illness." —Miss D. M.[9]

Dr. Benjamin Lau reports the case of two sisters from Singapore who came to the United States for their college educations.[10] During their second year in Los Angeles they both developed symptoms of hay fever—sneezing, streamy nasal discharge, and watery itching eyes. The antihistamines prescribed by their physician brought some relief but caused many unpleasant side effects including the inability to concentrate. Desensitized shots were administered after skin tests indicated multiple allergies, but had little or no effect.

The parents, deeply concerned about their daughters' conditions contacted Dr. Lau and asked for his help. Dr. Lau told the two sisters they could have their choice, either acupuncture or Kyolic® Formula 102. After one acupuncture treatment, both girls said they'd rather try the garlic formula (acupuncture treatments involve some pain).

Dr. Lau instructed each girl to take 6 capsules of Kyolic® Formula 102 every day. Within 3 weeks both were free of hay fever symptoms. That was several years ago.

One of the sisters has remained in California and takes Kyolic® garlic capsules only when the area in which she lives becomes heavy with smog. The other sister returns to California every year to visit family members. Although she is free of hay fever all year while in Singapore, the moment she gets off the plane in Los Angeles she begins to sneeze. She quickly controls the problem by immediately taking a few capsules of the Kyolic® Formula 102.

CARRAGEEN

Botanical Name: *Chondrus crispus*
Common Names: Irish Moss, Chondrus

Carrageen, commonly known as Irish moss, is a small perennial seaweed growing attached to submerged rocks beneath the level of low tide and beyond. In Europe it occurs in Norway, France, Spain, and the British Isles. In the Northwestern Atlantic it is found from New Jersy to Newfoundland.

The color of carrageen varies from yellowish-green to reddish-purple or brown depending on the season and other factors, such as the amount of light available (exposure to sunlight in shallow water to the shade of deeper water). When dried, it is considerably darker. This short, sturdy plant is repeatedly branched near the tips, the multiple branching giving it a crisp, tufted appearance somewhat resembling parsley.

Reported Uses of Carrageen

Carrageen is classed as demulcent, pectoral, mucilagenous, and nutritive. It is considered of value for colds, coughs, and bronchitis.

To prepare the decoction, 1 ounce of carrageen is added to 1-1/2 pints of boiling water, simmered gently for 15 minutes, and then strained. The juice of one lemon, a pinch of cinnamon, and a teaspoonful of honey is stirred into the decoction, and one teacupful is taken hot two or three times a day.

The same remedy may also be used with advantage during winter months as a preventive against colds when taken hot at bedtime and on cold mornings.

WILD PLUM

Botanical Name: *Prunus spinosa*
Common Name: Wild Plum Bark

The flowers of the wild plum bark are single or in pairs and very small compared to those of the domestic or garden plum. The wild species grows in Europe and Central China and appears in the United States in the double-flowered variety.

Remedial Uses

The antispasmodic action attributed to wild plum bark is said to be of considerable value for treating bronchitis and asthma. A tea made with 1 teaspoon of the cut, dried bark to 1 cup of boiling water. The cup is covered with a saucer, and the tea is allowed to stand until cold. It is then strained and reheated with a little honey added. One cupful is taken two or three times a day.

Case Studies

"I am using wild plum bark tea before bedtime and upon arising for my asthma and bronchitis. It certainly has been helping me. I have given this a long trial and can testify to the wonderful help received. Of course, right living and eating has also aided materially." —Mrs. S. B.

"I would not know what to do without wild plum bark for my chronic bronchitis. The plum bark tea loosens the terrible collection of mucus, enabling me to cough up the overnight's accumulation every morning. If it wasn't for the tea I would not be able to function." —Mr. F. L.

HOMEOPATHIC HERBAL REMEDIES

Following is a selection of homeopathic remedies for colds, influenza, and winter chills according to symptoms. They are used in the 6x potency (dosages on the bottles) obtainable from various health food stores and herb firms as well as pharmacies which manufacture and sell homeopathic products.

It is important to point out, however, that aconite, pulsatilla, and bryonia alba, though toxic in their crude form, are perfectly harmless when used in homeopathic preparations.

- *Allium cepa* (Red Onion)

Streaming cold. Profuse watery discharge from nose and eyes, headache. Frequent sneezing. Often a painful tearing cough: feels as if the cough will tear the larynx. Tickly cough. Rawness in the throat which quickly extends to the chest. Symptoms worse in a warm room and in the evening. Better in open air.

- *Aconitum* (Aconite)

The traditional homeopathic remedy for the early stages of a cold which develops suddenly from exposure to cold, dry wind. Where sudden chilliness has been followed by fever and there is restlessness, anxiety, sore throat, hoarse cough, and runny nose. Laryngitis. Condition worse at night. Great thirst for cold water.

- *Pulsatilla* (Wind Flower)

When the cold is firmly established. Catarrh. Nose stuffed up at night. Copious flow in the morning with thick, yellowy mucus. Worse in a warm room. The patient is emotionally touchy, peeved, and tearful. Enjoys being fussed over and craves sympathy.

- *Bryonia alba* (White Byrony)

The cold often begins in the nose. Sneezing, runny nose, rawness of the throat, aching eyes, and headache the first day; then the condition travels to the larynx, with hoarseness leading to bronchitis, and may end in pleurisy. Painful dry spasmodic cough. Cough with stitches in the chest, worse on breathing and coughing. Expectoration scanty. Aching in the limbs and back. Patient is irritable, thirsty for cold fluids, wants to lie still and be left alone.

This remedy is also used for influenza.

- *Eupatorium perfoliatum* (Boneset)

Intense aching in the bones, especially in the limbs and back. Fever. Headache with throbbing pain. Sore eyeballs. Hoarse voice. Cough worse at night. Patient can't stand being touched.

- *Capsicum annum* (Cayenne Pepper)

Sore throat with smarting pain. A shuddering chill after every drink of liquid. Throat is very red, discolored, purple, mottled, puffed. Cheeks and nose red and cold. Throat remains sore for a long time after a cold.

- *Euphrasia* (Eyebright Herb)

Bland nasal discharge. Indicated wherever strong eye symptoms are present (e.g., irritating eye discharge, margins of the lids red, swollen, and burning).

Dr. Dorothy Shepard mentions the beneficial effects of this remedy in cases of influenza epidemics. She says: "The temperature would drop in twenty-four hours, the eye trouble would disappear in thirty-six to forty-eight hours, and after a few days' rest in bed, on a diet of oranges, grapefruit and lemon juice, made from the fresh fruit, the patient would get up feeling like a new person."[11]

TRADITIONAL CHINESE HERB COMBINATIONS

There are numerous herbal formulas employed in traditional Chinese medicine for treating respiratory disorders. Following are a few examples of those most commonly used.

Pueraria Combination[12]

Constituents: Pueraria, ma-huang, cinnamon, paeonia, jujube, licorice, ginger.

Uses: This combination has been famous in China for its curative powers since ancient times. It is used for the common cold, influenza, bronchitis, and pneumonia.

The government of Japan has approved the Pueraria Combination for use in medical clinics for the common cold.

Minor Bupleurum Combination[13]

Constituents: Bupleurum, scute, pinellia, ginseng, jujube, licorice, ginger.

Uses: Taken for mild fever, cough, sticky phlegm, a bitter taste in the mouth, and a sensation of fullness in the chest. Also considered useful in conditions of acute or chronic bronchitis, asthma, pulmonary emphysema, headache, nasal congestion, pneumonia, and the common cold accompanied by shoulder stiffness.

Minor Bupleurum Combination has been approved by the Japanese government for use in medical facilities for the common cold, other febrile diseases, bronchitis, pleurisy, and tuberculosis.

Pinellia and Magnolia Combination[14]

Constituents: Pinellia, magnolia bark, hoelen, ginger, perilla.

Uses: Considered effective for treating pleurisy, the common cold, influenza, pneumonia, and tuberculosis.

Bupleurum and Cinnamon Combination[15]

Constituents: Bupleurum, pinellia, licorice, cinnamon, scute, ginseng, paeonia, jujube, ginger.

Uses: Taken for pleurisy, a common cold, and a lingering cold with mild fever.

Hoelen and Schizandra Combination[16]

Constituents: Hoelen, schizandra, licorice, ginger, apricot seed, pinellia, asarum.

Uses: Traditional Chinese herbal practitioners consider this formula especially effective for treating chronic bronchitis or emphysema in the elderly or those of a delicate constitution.

The accompanying symptoms are poor complexion, asthmatic wheezing and cough, no energy, difficulty in breathing when climbing stairs, abdominal softness, and a cold.

Baked Licorice Combination[17]

Constituents: Baked licorice, jujube, ginger, ginseng, rehmannia, cinnamon, linum, ophiopogon, gelatin.

Uses: Baked Licorice Combination is given for chronic bronchitis, pulmonary emphysema, dry throat, shortness of breath, sputum difficult to dislodge, weak physique, and palpitations.

Licorice and Ma-Huang Combination[18]

Constituents: Licorice, ma-huang.

Uses: This combination is considered especially good for asthma, as the ephedrine in ma-huang eases coughing, convulsions, difficulty in breathing, and improves blood circulation. The licorice reputedly removes the toxins that cause asthma.

Note. Traditional Chinese herb formulas are available on the market. Check with herb firms.

Case Studies

A correspondent writes: "The product called Hoelen and Schizandra has helped my husband with his emphysema condition *so much* that I will continue giving it to him.

"This morning his doctor told me he is doing so well that he need not have the usual check of X-ray for his lungs. Isn't that wonderful!" —Mrs. L. H. S.

Dr. Terashi cites the following case:[19] "Since the age of four, a forty year old man had suffered from asthma. It turned very serious during his second and third years of primary school, especially from September to December. However, between the ages of twenty and twenty-eight he experienced no attacks; at that time he lived in a different area of Japan. Many physicians had seen him over the years but none could help. Once again, though, the attacks were recurring. Of an average physique, he was thirsty and craved tea, water, and spices. Abdominal examination revealed chest distress. He took Minor Bupleurum Combination with Pinellia and Magnolia Combination for four months. His physical condition improved and he experienced no recurrence of asthma during the fall and winter."

SUMMARY

1. Coltsfoot herb has an ancient reputation as a remedy for loosening mucus and relieving irritation and persistent coughing in conditions of lung and bronchial ailments.
2. Soviet research teams have demonstrated that the herb eleuthero has an antiinfluenzal effect.
3. Yerba Santa has been effectively used from past to present for treating certain respiratory complaints.
4. Iceland moss is highly recommended by herbalists for relieving colds, coughs, hoarseness, and bronchitis.

5. Inhaling an essence of ginkgo helps to cure the common cold according to a medical specialist.

6. Garlic is a miracle remedy that may be used in different ways for treating a host of respiratory ailments.

7. A decoction of carrageen may be used with advantage for treating coughs, colds, and bronchitis. It is also helpful in preventing the common cold when used during the winter months.

8. Because of its antispasmodic action, wild plum bark is considered a valuable remedy for relieving asthma and bronchitis.

9. Homeopathic herbal remedies for treating colds, influenza, and winter chills are welcome additions to the family medicine cabinet.

10. Certain traditional Chinese herb formulas are used for treating asthma, emphysema, bronchitis, and other respiratory disorders.

11. When using any herbal remedy for respiratory ailments, other health practices should also be adopted (e.g., proper diet, fresh air, sufficient rest, nutritional supplements).

ENDNOTES

1. Hong-Yen Hsu Ph.D., "Chinese Herb Therapy for Asthma," *Bulletin of the Oriental Healing Arts Institute*, Vol. 6, No. 6, 1981.

2. L. A. Gagarin, *Adaptations and Adaptogens* (Vladivostok: The Far Eastern Scientific Center, USSR Academy of Sciences, 1977).

3. I. I. Brekhman, *Eleutherococcus* (Moscow: Uneshtorgizdat, 1977).

4. *Grace*, Autumn, 1982.

5. Ibid., Summer 1979.

6. *Hamburger Abendblatt*, October 8, 1966.

7. Tim Friend, *USA Today*, June 7, 1988.

8. J. H. Oliver, *Proven Remedies* (London: Thorsons Publishers Ltd.).

9. *Grace*, Autumn 1972.

10. Benjamin Lau, M.D., Ph.D., *Garlic for Health* (Wilmot, WI: Lotus Light Publications, 1988).

11. *A Physicians's Posy* (Rustington, Sussex, England: Health Science Press, 1969).

12. Dr. Hong-Yen Hsu, D. H. Easer, *Major Chinese Herbal Formulas* (Long Beach, CA: Oriental Healing Arts Institute, 1980).

13. Ibid.

14. Ibid.

15. Ibid.

16. Bokuso Terashi, M.D., *The Problems of Aging*, translated by Dr. Hong-Yen Hsu (Long Beach, CA: Oriental Healing Arts Institute, 1984).

17. Ibid.

18. Ibid.

19. Ibid.

CHAPTER 11

HERBAL AIDS FOR NERVOUS TENSION, INSOMNIA, AND HEADACHES

Some years ago, singer Debbie Boone reportedly experienced severe bouts of nervousness when performing on television. According to the news article,[1] Debbie said, "My hands would get so shaky that sometimes I couldn't even sign my name. I'd get stomach aches, headache and insomnia." She added that sometimes she'd tremble so much she could not even hold a microphone.

Debbie recalled the first time she ever appeared on the Dinah Shore show with her sister. She had the lead vocal, and for the first half of the song she was in control of her nervousness. But then "something hit me like 'I guess this is it—we're on the air,'" she said. "My face started twitching. I wanted to run off so bad—but there was no running. When the song was over I was trembling and then they broke for a commercial. I took a deep breath."

Ever since the young singer visited a nutritionalist she reported that her nervous disorders became less serious and less frequent. "The nutritionalist gave me herbs," she explained, "little herb pills called Calms Forté—that I take before a real stressful situation such as the Academy Awards or the Grammys. The herbs are not addictive and you can buy them at the health food store. I did get a lot calmer. The herbs balance my nervous system and the effects I get from being nervous, such as the quiver in my voice, go away."

Along with using the Calms Forté herb tablets, Debbie said she has eliminated processed food from her diet and now eats fresh vegetables, fruits, fowl, fish, and fresh whole grain products.

As a result of the herbal and nutritional program, she reported that she has felt so calm that she actually fell asleep during a talk show. "I was on the Dinah Shore show and some guy was reading poetry," she said. "I sat there and put my hand on my chin and fell asleep! Now that's certainly a good transition from the way I used to be."

What Is Calms Forté?

This is a homeopathic formula consisting of four natural herbal extracts in tablet form for nervous tension and insomnia, fortified with the five biochemic phosphates (calcium, iron, potassium, magnesium, and sodium) for nerve and brain fatigue.

As a relaxant, one to two tablets are taken three times daily, preferably before meals. For insomnia, take one to three tablets, half an hour to an hour before retiring. If needed, the tablets can be repeated, as there reportedly is no danger of side effects.

The herbal extracts contained in the Calms Forté product are passion flower, oats, hops, and chamomile. Let us examine these four plants as well as some of the others which have been effectively used in herbal medicine for treating nervous tension, sleeplessness, and headaches.

PASSION FLOWER

Botanical Name: *Passiflora incarnata*
Common Names: Passion Vine, Maypops, Purple Passion Flower

Most species of passion flower are native to the West Indies, South America, and the southern part of the United States. In their native habitat these vines often reach the tops of the tallest trees, where they sustain themselves by means of tendrils and send out an abundance of luxuriant blossoms. The flowers are almost white except for the purple center and blue or pink calyx crown. This handsome climber is one of the most graceful and lovely plants and can be used for covering trellises and arbors.

The Flower of Passion

The early Spanish missionaries in America were the first to call passiflora the "flower of passion," as they saw in it a representation of some of the objects associated with the Crucifixion. A description and drawing of the plant sent to Rome caused great excitement among botanists and theologians, as it was thought to be a wonderful illustration of the Cross triumphant in the world of Nature. Shortly after, the plant was introduced into Spain and Italy, and some remarkable specimens were soon produced in gardens of horticulturists. "This wonderful plant," wrote Aldinus, a Cardinal's physician, "is celebrated by poets, reasoned about by philosophers, praised by physicians for its numberless virtues, wondered about by theologians and venerated by Christians."

The Mystical Interpretation of Passion Flower

The early Spanish missionaries attributed the following symbolism to passion flower.

The column rising from the center of the flower represents the upright beam of the Cross. Above this are three small stems indicating the nails which pierced the Savior's hands and feet. Surmounting the column is the corona, symbolizing the crown of thorns, and around it is a veil of fine hairs, 72 in number, which are said to correspond to the number of thorns of which the crown was composed. The tendrils are suggestive of the cords and whips, while the small seed vessel is the sponge filled with vinegar which was offered to quench the Lord's thirst. The five deep red spots on each of the leaves are the five wounds.

When the flower is not entirely open, it resembles a star and represents the Star of the East seen by the Three Wise Men. The five petals and five sepals indicate the 10 apostles (Peter, who denied the Lord, and Judas, who betrayed him, are omitted). The purple color inside the blossom is the purple robe which was put on Christ in mockery. The white blossoms represent the purity and brightness of the Son of God.

The flowers grow singly on the stem, typifying the loneliness of Christ. The leaves are set on the stock singly, for there is one God, but are triplicate in form to testify to the Trinity. The plant is a vine and requires support, so the Christian who would aspire needs Divine assistance. The bell shape assumed by the flower when opening and fading means that God has not chosen to reveal the mysteries of His power until such time as His infinite Wisdom deems best. If the plant is cut down, it readily grows again; therefore, the person who loves God cannot be harmed by the evil in the world.

Such was the symbolism attributed to the plant by the Spanish missionaries, and to this day the flower still retains much of its religious associations.

Medicinal Uses of Passion Flower

Passion flower is classed as sedative, nervine, and antispasmodic. Dr. LeClerc of Paris showed that it has a calming effect on nervous restlessness, especially during convalescence, and that its use neither results in disorientation nor depression. Dr. Neiderkorn of Lloyd's pharmaceutical company found that it tones the sympathetic nervous system in asthenic (weakened) conditions, improving the circulation and nutrition of the nerve centers.

In a British publication,[2] Dr. Eric Powell writes:

> Why resort to drugs when a harmless plant like passion flower will produce the desired results, and without harm? This precious plant has been described as the remedy that brings peace to mind and body. Acting through the brain and nervous system it relaxes where there is muscular or organic tension, eases pain (pain is always associated with tension and contraction) and promotes a state of calmness throughout the entire organism. We have found it is of great value in spasmodic conditions, nervous headaches, neuralgia, hysteria and high blood pressure when due to nervous causes. What is not generally known is the it is an eye tonic, and a very good one.

Methods of Using Passion Flower

Passion Flower may be used alone in the form of a tincture, 15 to 60 drops in a little water, repeated as needed. However, it is more effective when combined with other herbs of similar properties. For example:

Tincture of passion flower: 1 oz.

Tincture of skullcap: 1 oz.

The two tinctures are mixed together, and 20 to 60 drops are taken in water as required.

Passion flower is also available on the market as one of the ingredients in professionally prepared herbal combinations, such as the product Calms Forté.

OATS

Botanical Name: *Avena sativa*
Common Name: Common Oat

Oats are grasses cultivated for their cereal grain. The stem is rough, with pale green leaves, and reaches up to 4 feet high. If the whole husk of the oat is removed the result is groats; if the grains are passed between heated rollers the result is rolled oats; the grains crushed in coarse or fine powder become oatmeal.

Remedial Uses of Oats

Oats are one of the most nutritious cereals, of particular value in special diets for convalescents. In herbal medicine they are classed as nervine, antispasmodic, and stimulant.

As a restorative and tonic, a fluid extract or tincture of oats strengthens yet calms the nerves in conditions of nervous prostration and insomnia. As an antispasmodic, it quickly relieves spasms of the ureter and bladder.

The dose of the tincture is 10 to 20 drops three times a day in water; of the fluid extract, 10 to 30 drops. When taken in hot water, the fluid extract becomes a stimulant.

HOPS

Botanical Name: *Humulus lupulus*
Common Name: Hops

The hop vine is native to the United States and Europe but has been found growing wild in many other parts of the world. It is a twining perennial plant which attaches itself to neighboring objects and climbs to a great height. In hop districts the plants are grown on long poles.

Hops are largely cultivated in many countries for their cones and strobiles, which are used in the manufacture of beer and ale.

Hop Pillow: Nature's Sleep Aid

Hop pickers of yesteryear claimed that the strong odor of hops exerted a soothing influence on the nerves and produced drowsiness. It was also claimed that many instances occurred in which people entering an "oast house" where hops were being dried, experienced such a relaxing effect that they felt compelled to sit down, and soon found themselves drifting off into a sound sleep.

Pillows stuffed with hops were soon used in place of ordinary pillows to insure a good night's sleep for sufferers of insomnia. This folk practice was considered superstitious nonsense until a hop pillow was prescribed for King George III in 1787 with excellent results. Records also show that it was employed with success during an illness suffered by the Prince of Wales in 1879.

The Hop Pillow in Modern Times

To this day, hop pillows have retained their popularity for allaying restlessness and producing sleep in nervous disorders. Scientific research has shown that hops contain certain substances which act as a sedative in overcoming insomnia. Lupulin, the active ingredient in hops, has been used with good effect in war psychosis.

A hop pillow is prepared by filling a small muslin bag loosely with hops and attaching it to an ordinary pillow. Some people sprinkle the hops with a little alcohol, claiming that it helps to enhance the sedative properties.

The Remedial Value of Hop Tea

Hops are classified as nervine, soporific, anodyne, stomachic, and tonic.

Hop tea is prescribed for sleeplessness, hysteria, nervous irritability, and nervous sick headache. It is also employed in dyspepsia and debility.

The tea is prepared with 1 ounce of hops to 1 pint of boiling water. The container is covered with a lid, and the tea is simmered for two or three minutes and then removed from the burner and allowed to stand for five minutes. It is then strained.

In conditions of insomnia and nervous irritation, one hot teacupful is sipped two or three times a day and once before bedtime. For nervous sick headache, a teacupful every three hours is taken; during a severe attack, every two hours. (Hop tea has an extremely bitter taste and may be sweetened with honey.)

CHAMOMILE

Botanical Name: *Matricaria chamomilla*
Common Names: German Chamomile, Chamomilla

German chamomile is an annual plant indigenous to Southern Europe, found growing wild in fields, meadows, and along roadsides. When cultivated in gardens, the stems are upright, about a foot high, hollow, furrowed and downy, but in a wild state they are prostrate. The yellow or whitish flower heads of German chamomile are much smaller than those of the Roman variety.

This plant is said to be consecrated to St. Anne, the Mother of the Virgin Mary, seemingly because of the herb's botanical name, *Matricaria*, which is derived from *mater* and *cara*, meaning "beloved mother."

Remedial Uses

German chamomile is classed as sedative, anodyne, carminative, and tonic. It has a well-established reputation as a remedy for soothing the nerves, strengthening digestion, and relieving certain forms of colic. The tea is a popular beverage in European countries, where it is taken at bedtime for conditions of insomnia. The tea is also widely accepted as a domestic remedy for the treatment of nightmare and restless sleep, especially in children. An English physician, Dr. Schall, claimed the tea was not only an effective remedy for nightmare but was also an excellent preventive of this complaint.

The tea is prepared by placing 2 teaspoons of the dried flower heads in a cup and adding boiling water. The cup is immediately covered with a saucer, and the tea is allowed to stand for 5 or 10 minutes before straining off. One or two teacups may be taken daily, a mouthful at a time. For insomnia, a half-cup is taken at bedtime. The amount for children is 1 or 2 tablespoons two or three times a day.

FEVERFEW

Botanical Name: *Tanacetum parthenium*
Common Names: Headache Plant, Febrifuge Plant

There are several variations of feverfew, but the more common wild variety is known as *Tanacetum parthenium*. It is a native of Europe but is also found growing in the fields and waysides in many parts of North America. This aromatic plant bears clusters of daisy-like flowers with yellow central disks and white petals. The leaves are green with a touch of yellow.

Early Medicinal Uses

The word *feverfew* is a corruption of *febrifuge* (lowers fever), which indicates the idea dating from earliest times that the plant was effective for treating elevated body temperature. It was also employed for a number of other ailments including headaches, dizziness, and arthritis. John Gerard, in his famous *Herball* (1597), wrote "Feverfew dried and made into powder, and two drams of it taken with honey or sweet wine dispels melancholy and phlegm; there it is good for those that are 'giddie in the head,' or who have the turning called vertigo—that is, a swimming in the head." In his *Family Herbal* (1772), Dr. John Hill stated, "In the worst headache, this herb (feverfew) exceeds whatever else is known."

Among the early colonists feverfew was used to treat chills, fever, and headache pain.

Modern Usage

Feverfew is classed as febrifuge, diaphoretic, carminative, antipyretic, and tonic.

In modern England, some people who have found the usual migraine treatments ineffective have been eating two to four feverfew leaves a day as a familiar method of preventing migraine headache attacks. Generally, the leaves are eaten between two slices of bread or with other food to mask their bitter taste.

To evaluate the remedy, a group of British medical researchers began a series of clinical studies. However, before presenting the details of some of these reports, let us consider a few facts about migraine headaches.

Migraine

The word *migraine* is translated from the Greek, meaning "half the skull," as the excruciating pain usually strikes one side of the head. Scientists use the term *dols* as a measurement of pain. On a chart, six dols is given as the degree of pain the average person seldom exceeds. Intense migraine headache is listed at nine.

Between eight and twelve million Americans periodically suffer from this distressing condition, and victims are very familiar with the warning signs of an impending attack. Vision distortion is common as things begin to look blurry or hazy. Black spots or flickering, flashing lights may appear before the eyes. The victim may also feel dizzy. Shortly thereafter, a throbbing, pounding sensation of pain is experienced on one side of the head, concentrated over the right eye, but with some people it occurs over the left.

The pain quickly reaches its full fury and in some cases may eventually extend to the crown of the head. To compound the misery, a migraine attack is often accompanied by nausea and vomiting. When this occurs, the patient's face is usually drawn, pale, and haggard, the eyes sunken.

Some Possible Causes of Migraine

According to various medical opinions, some of the possible causes of migraine are:

- Glandular deficiencies, a conclusion based on the fact that migraine attacks often cease in middle age when gland functions slow down—with women at the time of menopause, and with men in their fifties.
- Forms of mental tension such as grief, anxiety, rage, shattering disappointments, and persistent worrying thoughts.
- Constipation with resulting autointoxication.
- Allergy due to one or more foods, or food preservatives. Some examples are cheese, milk, wheat, pork, chocolate, beer, and wine, which have been linked to migraine. Dietary restriction of foods suspected of causing migraine headache has eliminated or relieved the problem in 50% of the cases studied.
- Wrong eating habits. The two most common faults are inadequate breakfast and an excess of carbohydrates. The diet should be low fat, high protein, and medium carbohydrate.
- Inhalants and certain odors can start the cycle that results in throbbing, blinding headaches for susceptible persons. The most common among the offending inhalants are house dust and mold; the odors are smog, paint, paint thinners, perfumes, frying odors, aerosols, motor exhaust, ammonia, chlorine, and formaldehyde (a chemical used in some of the stay-press garments and in most sheets and pillow cases).
- Liver trouble. Normally the bile which forms in the liver cells is thin and clear and flows freely through the bile

ducts. But if it thickens, generally due to consumption of fatty foodstuffs or temporary congestion of the bile ducts, the flow is sluggish and may cause the bile to back up into the bloodstream. This can result in the type of migraine headache referred to by such terms as *liverish migraine headache, sick headache, bilious sick headache*. Symptoms generally include nausea and the vomiting of greenish-yellow bile. In this condition it is important that attention be given to the health of the liver (refer to chapter 2).

Scientific Studies on the Use of Feverfew

Researchers in Great Britain are reporting success with the use of feverfew, not only in reducing fever and arthritic inflammation but especially in preventing or relieving migraine headaches. For example, in October 1978, the first of a series of articles was published in *The Lancet*, a prestigious medical journal. The article stated that more than "70% of 270 migraine sufferers who have eaten feverfew leaves every day for prolonged periods claimed that the herb decreased the frequency of the attacks or caused them to be less painful or both." The success rate was considered remarkably high in view of the fact that most of the patients had not responded to orthodox medical treatment.

About 18% of the feverfew users suffered undesirable side effects, usually soreness of the tongue or mouth.

Other articles on the use of fewerfew soon followed. Then later, the results of a study conducted at the City of London Migraine Clinic were published in an issue of the *British Medical Journal*.[3] The aim of the study was to recruit 20 patients who had been eating feverfew leaves of their own accord every day for at least three months as a means of reducing their migraine headache attacks. The test was designed in which feverfew would be withdrawn from 10 of the patients by giving them a placebo, while the other 10 would receive 50 milligrams of freeze-dried powdered feverfew leaves daily in capsule form.

Three of the patients refused to participate, as they were fearful of a return in the frequency or severity of their migraine attacks if they were assigned to the group not getting the feverfew capsules. Of the 17 patients, eight were given freeze-dried feverfew, and nine received the placebo. Neither group knew which treatment they were getting, as the placebo and feverfew were presented in identical capsules.

The result of the study showed that among those taking the placebo, the nausea, vomiting, and frequency of the attacks virtually tripled. In comparison, patients given the feverfew capsules suffered no change in the frequency of the attacks and they had far fewer and less severe headaches. The researchers concluded that "this provides evidence that feverfew taken prophylactically, prevents attacks of migraine."

Another study on the use of feverfew in migraine prevention was conducted at the Department of Medicine, University Hospital, Nottingham.[4] Following is the abstract/summary:

The use of feverfew (*Tanacetum parthenium*) for migraine prophylaxis was assessed in a randomized double-blind, placebo-controlled crossover study. After a one month single-blind placebo run-in, 72 volunteers were randomly allocated to receive either one capsule of dried feverfew leaves a day or matching placebo for four months and then transferred to the other treatment limb for a further four months. Frequency and severity of attacks were determined from diary cards which were issued every two months; efficacy of each treatment was also assessed by visual analogue scores. 60 patients completed the study and full information was available in 59. Treatment with feverfew was associated with a reduction in the mean number and severity of attacks in each two-month period, and in the degree of vomiting; duration of individual attacks was unaltered. Visual analogue scores also indicated a significant improvement with feverfew. There were no serious side effects.

Scientific Evaluation of Feverfew

From their studies, scientists have ascertained that extracts of feverfew inhibit the production of prostaglandins, substances believed responsible for the constriction and dilation of blood vessels of the brain which occur in attacks of migraine. The extracts also inhibited release of seratonin, which may contribute to migraine. Inhibition of PMNs (polymorphonuclear leucocytes), granules found in the lubricating fluid of the joints in conditions of arthritis, was also established. Vitamin B_{12}-binding protein produced from PMNs is inhibited as well.

Feverfew has a different effect on platelets (certain constituents in the blood) and is more pronounced that other nonsteroid, noninflammatory agents such as aspirin. For example, it does not inhibit blood clotting.

Another healing component of feverfew is that of a phospholipase inhibitor, which accounts for its antifever and antiinflammatory activity.

Methods of Using Feverfew
as a Home Remedy

If the fresh or dried leaves are used, they should never be ingested by themselves but should be eaten with food (e.g., between two slices of bread or in a salad). The fresh plant may be obtained from herb nurseries.

The freeze-dried leaves are available in tablet or capsule form. Ideally, the label should state that the product contains no additives such as fillers, lubricants, or excipients.

Note. Feverfew should not be used during pregnancy or in conditions of allergies to plants of the ragweed family.

Case Studies Show Feverfew
Brings Migraine Relief

"From the time I was in my late twenties (I am 38 now), I suffered agonizing attacks of migraine headaches. But thank the good Lord, I have been healed by eating one large feverfew leaf daily for the past three years, and there have been no further migraine attacks in all that time." —R. C.

"I have tried numerous medications for migraine headache, but nothing helped. Last year a woman I met in a health food store recommended feverfew tablets, 100 milligrams daily. I didn't think they'd do a bit of good, but I tried them anyway. Now I must admit to my surprise the migraine attacks are nowhere as bad or as often." —J. H.

"I am writing you about a treatment for overcoming distressing headache pain. Perhaps some other unfortunate person may be helped.

"My husband suffered frequent attacks of dreadful migraine headaches. The attacks became much less severe and less frequent after he gave up eating cheese. A naturopathic doctor explained that cheddar cheese, beer, and some wines contain a substance called tyramine, which can cause migraine in susceptible people.

"Although greatly relieved, my husband was not completely cured until he heard about an herb called feverfew; the botanical name is *Tanacetum parthenium*. He took capsules of the leaves every day until his headaches completely disappeared. He found, however, that he could not return to eating cheese again. The treatment only worked for him if he took the feverfew capsules and avoided eating cheese." —Mrs. B. C.

A man and his wife said they found feverfew to be of tremendous value for anyone suffering from migraine headaches. They noticed improvement after approximately two months of eating a sandwich of the leaves every morning. Improvement was total after six months.

Proof of the effectiveness of feverfew was evident when they lost their plants in the winter. Within three weeks their migraine headaches returned. Later when they were able to resume eating their feverfew sandwiches, they felt immediate improvement.

FRINGE TREE

Botanical Name: *Chionanthus virginicus*
Common Names: American Fringe Tree, Snow Flowers, Old Man's Beard, White Fringe

Fringe tree is considered an excellent remedy for the type of headache commonly called liverish migraine. It may be taken in the form of a fluid extract, 1/2 to 1 teaspoon in a little water three times a day; or as a tincture, 10 to 15 drops in water three times daily.

There have been instances where some migraine sufferers who did not obtain results from using the tincture or extract were reportedly cured by taking the remedy in homeopathic form. The tiny pellets were taken in the 6x potency according to directions on the bottles.

In addition to taking the fringe tree remedy in any form, victims of liverish migraine are advised to avoid eating or drinking anything cold. All foods or fluids should be warm or hot.

Fried foods and dairy products such as cream, milk, eggs, butter, and cheese are to be omitted from the diet. If irregularity is a problem, steps should be taken to keep the bowels open.

ROSE HIPS

Rose hips are the fruit of the rose after the flower has blossomed and the petals have fallen, just as the cherry is the fruit of the cherry blossom. They are orange in color when not quite ripe, dark red when overripe, and bright red when fully ripe.

The ancient Greeks in the time of Homer made a food of rose hips, and a thousand years before the birth of Christ the hips were referred to as the Food of the Gods. Gods were believed to be men who lived so close to Nature that she whispered all her secrets to them.

Rose Hips Vitamin C for Migraine Headache

Some people have found relief from migraine headaches with the use of rose hips vitamin C tablets. For example, P. C. writes:[5] "I never knew what it was like to go through a whole month without a murderous buzz-saw biting into the left side of my skull. How did I get relief? It came by taking three 100 milligram tablets of Rose Hip vitamin C. At first I couldn't believe it. There are many causes of migraine, and as many cures. But this is what it did for me."

Another case was that of Mr. D. P., who described his experience in a letter to the *London Daily Telegraph*. He wrote: "I had a severe migraine attack when it was necessary for me to do a lot of driving. In desperation I swallowed five 50 milligram vitamin C tablets. Much to my surprise, the flashing lights and 'saw-edged' patterns disappeared within minutes and with no subsequent headache."

Mr. P. went on to say, "I think there are probably many cases of migraine and there are probably other people who find it (vitamin C) helpful. My doctor's reaction was that it could 'do no harm' and he was completely skeptical."

As a result of his letter, Mr. P. received many correspondences from his readers. He said, "This included two or three people who have thanked me, saying their attacks have ceased within 30 minutes. I think it is also significant that grapefruit and grapefruit juice are effective. But orange juice has the opposite and makes the attacks worse. One of my correspondents has also found that lemon juice is helpful. Could it be that migraine is associated with a liver disorder?"

Note. It seems apparent from Mr. P.'s question that he was aware of lemon juice being an old-time remedy for liver trouble. The juice has been employed in a variety of ailments including liverish migraine headaches.

SKULLCAP

Botanical Name: *Scutellaria laterifolia*
Common Names: Mad Dogweed, Hoodwort, Blue Skullcap

Skullcap is indigenous to North America, growing in damp places alongside ponds and in meadows from Connecticut south to Florida and Texas. It reaches about 3 feet in height, with small flowers of a pale blue color.

The plant was given the common name of mad dogweed, as it was considered in olden times to be a remedy for hydrophobia.

Modern Uses

Skullcap is considered an effective nerve tonic, exerting a soothing and calming influence on the cerebrospinal system, allaying hysterical excitement, inner tension, and restlessness. It is also helpful for nervous headaches.

An infusion is prepared by adding 1 ounce of the herb to 1 pint of boiling water. The container is immediately removed from the burner, covered with a lid, and allowed to stand until lukewarm. It is then strained and taken in half teacupful doses every few hours.

For insomnia, skullcap is generally combined with other herbs. Here is a formula that has worked well for some people:

> Equal parts of skullcap, peppermint, and catnip are thoroughly mixed together. One or two teaspoons of the mixture are placed in a cup, and boiling water added. The cup is covered with a saucer, and the tea is allowed to stand until lukewarm and is then strained. One warm cupful is taken at night before retiring.

WOOD BETONY

Botanical Name: *Betonica Officianalis*
Common Names: Betony, Bishopwort, Betonic

Wood betony is a European plant found growing in shady woods and meadows, reaching a height of from 6 inches to 2 feet. It bears purple-red flowers arranged on whorls at the top of the stems. The leaves are cordate, oblong, their surface dotted with glands containing an aromatic oil.

Betonic is the Celtic name of the plant and comes from *ben* (the head) and *ton* (good) in allusion to the herb's virtues as a remedy for head complaints.

Early Uses

Antonius Musa, physician to Augustus Caesar, valued the plant as an effective remedy in no less than 47 diseases, and Culpeper remarked that "It was not the practice of Caesar to keep fools about him."

An early herbarium written by Apuleius stated that betony is "good whether for a man's soul or for his body; it shields him against frightful visions and dreams, and the wort is very wholesome." The following statement appears in the *Medicina Britannica*, 1666: "I have known the worst obstinate headaches cured by daily breakfasting for a month or six weeks on a decoction of Betony made with new milk and strained." Turner, in his *British Physician*, 1687, wrote: "It would seem a miracle to tell what experience I have had with it (betony), not only in cases of insomnia but in removing pain from any part of the head."

At one time wood betony was used as an ingredient in snuff as a headache remedy.

Modern Uses

Wood betony is used for the relief of nervous headache, migraine headaches, and insomnia by placing two heaping teaspoons of the dried herb in a cup and adding boiling water. This is allowed to cool and is then strained. One-half teacupful is taken morning and evening or more often in severe cases.

Betony is said to be more effective when combined with other herbs of similar properties. For example:

Wood betony: 2 oz.

Rosemary: 1 oz.

Skullcap: 1 oz.

After thoroughly mixing, one-quarter of the mixture is placed in 1 pint of cold water and brought to a boil, simmered for two minutes, strained, and allowed to stand until cold.

One teacup is taken three times daily. For insomnia an extra teacup of the beverage is taken hot at bedtime.

SUMMARY

1. The four herbal extracts contained in the Calms Forté product are passion flower, oats, hops, and chamomile.
2. Passion flower is classed as sedative, nervine, and antispasmodic and described as bringing peace to mind and body.
3. A fluid extract or tincture of oats strengthens yet calms the nerves in conditions of nervous prostration and insomnia.
4. A tea of hops is used for sleeplessness, nervous irritability, hysteria, and nervous sick headache.
5. A pillow of hops is popular for relieving restlessness and producing sleep in nervous disorders.

6. Chamomile is soothing to the nerves and has a well-deserved reputation a remedy for insomnia. It is also valued
for the treatment of restless sleep and nightmare, especially in children.

7. There are many causes of migraine headache, the most
common resulting from liver trouble. It is referred to by
such terms as liverish migraine, sick headache, and bilious sick headache.

8. In liversish migraine it is important that attention be
given to the health of the liver.

9. Many scientific studies have shown that feverfew not
only reduces fever and arthritic inflammation but also
prevents or relieves migraine headaches.

10. If fresh or dried feverfew leaves are used, they should
never be ingested by themselves but should be eaten with
food.

11. Products containing freeze-dried feverfew in tablet or
capsule form are available on the market.

12. Feverfew should not be used during pregnancy or where
there are allergies to plants of the ragweed family.

13. Fringe tree is considered especially valuable as a remedy
for liverish migraine headache.

14. Some migraine sufferers have benefitted from the use of
fringe tree in fluid extract or tincture form, whereas others
have found that the homeopathic form of fringe tree works
best for them.

15. Rose hips vitamin C has brought relief from migraine
headaches for some people.

16. Skullcap is valued as an effective nerve tonic and as a
remedy for relieving nervous headaches, migraine headaches, and insomnia.

ENDNOTES

1. B. Bert, *National Enquirer*, July 18, 1978.
2. *Fitness and Health From Herbs*, March 1964.
3. August 31, 1985.
4. *The Lancet*, July 23, 1988.
5. *Health Digest*, Vol. 1, No. 3, 1971.

MAIL ORDER HERB DEALERS

Kwan Yin Herb Company, Inc.
P.O. Box 18617
Spokane, WA 99208
(Chinese and Domestic Herbs)

Golden Gate Herbs, Inc.
P.O. Box 890
Forestville, CA 95436

Nature's Herb Company
1010 46th St.
Emeryville, CA 94608

Hausmann's Pharmacy
534-536 W. Girard Ave.
Philadelphia, PA 19123

Indiana Botanical Gardens
P.O. Box 5
Hammond, IN 46325

Penn Herb Company
603 North 2nd St.
Philadelphia, PA 19123

Pacific Trends, Inc.
21520 Blythe St.
Canoga Park, CA 91304

IN CANADA
Nu-Life Nutrition, Ltd.
871 Beatty St.
Vancouver, B.C., Canada

INDEX

A

Abdominal pain, and pinellia and ginseng six combination, 113
Abscesses: and echinacea, 96-97, 142
and honey, 93-94
and slippery elm, 142-43
Acne: and garlic, 15
and lemon, 138
and propolis, 145-46
Aconite, 164
Acquired Immune Deficiency Syndrome (AIDS), 2
and garlic, 14, 16-17
and Kyolic™, 17
and minor bupleurum combination, 20
and shiitake, 9
Acute respiratory diseases (ARD), and eleuthero, 156-57
Adaptogens, definition of, 3
Agnus castus, 43-45, 83-84, 87
case studies of use, 44-45
and genitourinary problems, 83-84
for male disorders, 84
mechanism of, 44
and osteoporosis, 67-68
remedial uses of, 43
scientific evaluation of, 43-44
AIDS, See Acquired Immune Deficiency Syndrome (AIDS)
Alisma, 114
Allantoin, 90, 102
Allergy, 2
and migraine headaches, 179
and reishi, 7
Aloe vera, 100-101, 102
case studies of use, 101
medicinal uses of, 100
methods of use, 100-101
Alzheimer's disease, 118-20, 134
and aluminum, 118-20, 135
combatting, 119-20
See also Memory deterioration
Amenorrhea, 42, 45, 47
American elm, See Slippery elm
American fringe tree, See Fringe tree
Anemia, 2
Anorexia: and pinellia combination, 113
and six major herb combination, 115

Antibody production, 2
Antigens, definition of, 3
Anxiety:
and hawthorn, 124
See also Nervous tension
Apple cider vinegar, 151
as a deodorant, 148
and skin problems, 147-48
Apricot seed, 166
Apricot seed and linum combination formula, 114
Arberry, See Uva-ursi
Areca seed, 49
Arthritis: and chaparral, 55-60
and cherry, 68-70
and eleuthero, 5
and feverfew, 180
and garlic, 15
and yucca, 62-63
See also Rheumatism
Artichoke, 33-34
remedial uses, 34
scientific evaluation, 34
Asarum, 166
Ascites, and pipsissewa, 76-77
Asthma, 2
and coltsfoot, 156
and minor bupleurum combination, 165-66
symptoms of, 154
and wild plum, 163
and yerba santa, 157
Astragalus, 5-7, 20, 114
formulas, 6-7
modern uses, 5-6
traditional uses, 5
Astragalus Eight Herbs Formula, 6, 21
Atherosclerosis:
and ginseng, 130
and hawthorn, 124
Atherosclerotic dementia, 116
Athlete's foot:
and apple cider vinegar, 147-48
and garlic, 14-15
Atractylodes, 6, 48, 113, 114, 115

B

Baked licorice combination, 166
Balm, 45-46
medicinal uses, 46

D

E

H